FIT FOR LIFE
The Annapolis Way

A publication of
Leisure Press
P.O. Box 3; West Point, N.Y. 10996

Library of Congress Cataloging in Publication Data

Lenz, Heinz W.
    Fit for life.

    1. United States.   Navy—Physical training.
    2. United States Naval Academy—Athletics. 3. Physical
    fitness.   4. Physical education and training.
    I. Murray, John L.   II. Title
    V263.L46   1984   613.7'0088359   82-84099
    ISBN 0-88011-032-5

Athletic Photography by: Phil Hoffman, Naval Academy Photographer
Book Design/Production: David Hebenstreit

FIT FOR LIFE
The Annapolis Way

Heinz W. Lenz
Director of Personal Conditioning
U.S. Naval Academy

and

John L. Murray, PH. D.
Exercise Specialist

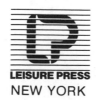

LEISURE PRESS
NEW YORK

To Ensign Alan W. Lenz, USN, Class of 1983, USNA, who trained hard to meet excellently the Academy's physical fitness requirements.

—HWL

To my mother and father, Emma Kathryn (Long) and John William Murray, for their unselfish love and encouragement.

—JM

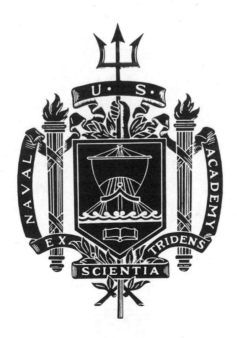

CONTENTS

ACKNOWLEDGMENTS

During the months of manuscript preparation many individuals enthusiastically and unselfishly contributed time, expertise and resources to the finished document. Their support was truly valued and sincere appreciation is extended to each of them.

Foremost we want to thank Dr. Jim Peterson, publisher of Leisure Press. Originally it was Jim's idea to create this book and it was his persistence which enabled us to move toward its completion.

We are indeed grateful to Commodore Leon A. Edney (USN, Commandant of Midshipmen), Captain J. O. "Bo" Coppedge, USN-ret, Commander Dave Church (USN, Executive Physical Education Officer) and Mr. Jim Gehrdes (Deputy Physical Education Officer) of the United States Naval Academy for their advice and encouragement throughout the project. Ed Wilson (USNA Publications Officer), Leo Mehalic (USNA Publications Office and the hat toss cover photographer), and Jack Moore (USNA Photo Laboratory) were always cordial hosts and graciously offered assistance any time it was requested.

Our special thanks go also to the members of the Personal Conditioning Committee (USNA) L. Greg Myers, Jan Dainard, Joseph Suriano, Cynthia J. Schendel, Robert Lawson, Barbara Lawson and Peter M. Kormann. We are especially grateful for Peter Kormann's efforts in developing the materials for the Muscular Fitness chapter.

For his creative and artistic ability as an athletic photographer we especially wish to recognize Phil Hoffman, USNA Athletic Association photographer, who was responsible for the athletic photographs used throughout the book. Ed Jathro (USNA Class of '72) contributed the PEP photographs. Furthermore, we want to acknowledge the assistance of the late Chick Wolszek, Athletic Association photographer, who gave us the idea of using historical athletic photographs in the book. Joan Sereboff also provided us with helpful suggestions and clerical assistance.

Appreciation is also extended to the individuals who willingly served as models for some of the photographs. Ensign Alan W. Lenz (USNA, Class of '83) was a perfect subject for the Nautilus training photographs. Dan Watts and Nancy Mullen were outstanding models for the flexibility chapter photographs.

Last and most importantly, we wish to express a very special thanks to our wives, Bette Lenz and Rae Murray, for their love, moral support, and unremitting patience. Despite many other family and professional obligations their encouragement enabled us to complete this project. Rae's expertise as a photographer and companion on the frequent trips to Annapolis made the task more enjoyable. And Bette's affable spirit provided the inspiration to make a dream become a reality.

FOREWORD

We must sail sometimes with the wind, sometimes against it; but we must sail and not drift or lie at anchor.

—Justice Oliver Wendell Holmes

Each commissioned officer bears an individual responsibility for maintaining a high standard of physical fitness. This commitment to a lifetime of physical fitness is more than a goal of long-term good health and a trim personal appearance; it is essential to military leadership. The physical fitness of a unit is directly related to combat readiness and the ability to perform under pressure. The leader who is physically fit not only sets the proper example for his subordinates, he is also more productive in his daily work environment in the Navy.

While the basic routine may be altered if your environment allows the luxury of space, the junior officer in the Navy should select a fitness routine that can be accomplished in a confined environment such as found aboard ship. In my twenty-five years of naval service, I have run three to five miles daily around the missile mount on a cruiser following sit-ups and deep knee bends in my stateroom, and I have run the same daily three to five miles on the deck of a carrier. The key to any exercise program is to make it a daily part of your schedule and then stick to it.

In addition to daily exercise, an essential part of every seagoing officer's fitness program must be a reasonable diet that varies the calorie intake with the amount of physical activity of the daily routine. This book points out several routines that are effective and have been successful. The key is to select one and stick to it. If you do, you will have that special extra energy and stamina when you need it, and you will be a better officer for this commitment to physical fitness.

Leon A. Edney, Commodore, USN
Commandant of Midshipmen
1979-83

PREFACE

Throughout the story of mankind physical strength and endurance along with personal courage have been common ingredients in survivability. In our rapidly changing and complex world we are rediscovering the importance of these human qualities. To exist in our worlds of tomorrow, our creative, intellectual, and spiritual energies can only be tapped when we are healthy and fit.

Personal fitness for military officers may mean survival. Maintaining personal fitness is an individual decision for each of us. We can choose to remain fit and strive toward a higher quality of existence, or we may choose to remain unfit and prematurely succumb to the ravages of our modern degenerative illnesses.

The first choice is filled with optimism, enthusiasm and a positive reverence for life. The second choice leads to pessimism, cynicism and a self-defeatist attitude.

In this book we hope to inspire and to persuade you to choose living fully and abundantly. Human life is too short and too precious a gift to view it otherwise.

The Authors

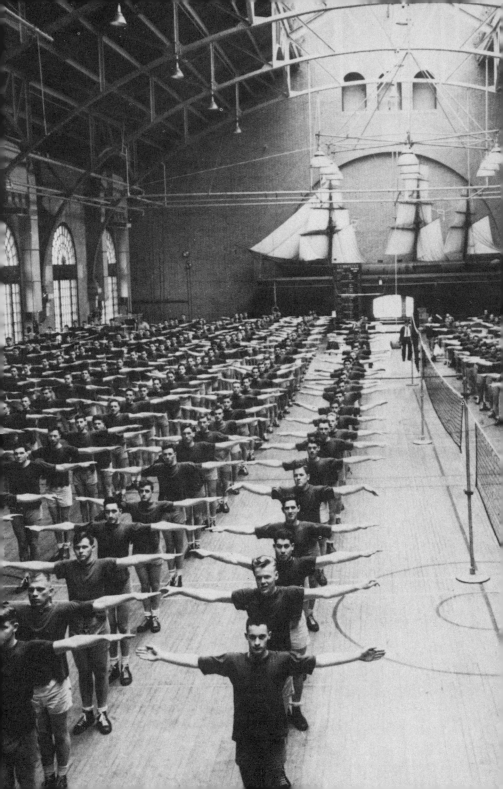

INTRODUCTION: FITNESS AND THE NAVY

FITNESS TRADITION

The U.S. Naval Academy has a rich tradition of requiring its future officers to undergo rigorous physical training. Although its beginnings were somewhat inauspicious and a mere distant cousin to the modern, sophisticated training and facilities currently used, the enthusiasm for and importance of such training was obvious even in 1867. Excerpts from a letter written by E.H.C. Leutze, Rear Admiral USN (Ret), give us an insight into the early program:

> During the summer of 1867 the Superintendent, Admiral D.D. Porter, reputed to be physically one of the most powerful officers of his time, filled in the deck of old Fort Severn as a Gymnasium. . . We did ground and loft tumbling, exercises and parallel and horizontal bars (including the Giant Swing), and exercises on trapezes. There were also drills with dumb-bells and Indian Clubs.

> Admiral Porter also had us lift heavy weights, such as a barrel of flour to our shoulders, a very difficult feat. In the Spring of 1867 we had the first boat race, between the First and Second classes, which the latter won . . . . There was also inter class baseball and old fashioned (Rugby) football.

> This to the best of my recollection after 60 years was the starting of athletics at the Academy.

MORAL, MENTAL AND PHYSICAL DEVELOPMENT

Experts in human development tell us that a quality of life is achieved by individuals who seek the development of a balanced personality. Although a variety of conceptual models have been used to illustrate personality traits, the three-dimensional model presented below represents the ideal development of a midshipman. For the men and women attending the U.S. Naval Academy the model symbolizes the importance of the physical, intellectual and moral components which together enable one to strive for a quality existence.

If a fully functional and healthy life is to be attained, all three sides of a person must be developed evenly. In contemporary society it appears that the more technologically advanced the society, the weaker the physical base becomes. At a great cost to humanity, we are learning that the physical base cannot be ignored. Instead, fitness training must be carried out by every man, woman and child to provide and maintain a strong physical foundation for a lifetime. Such a foundation will enable each of us to make the finest possible professional contribution in our chosen career. For individuals seeking a career in the military service, lifelong fitness training is essential.

At the U.S. Naval Academy, training closely embodies the three sides of the triangle. Daily throughout the four years of training, the total development of each midshipman is sought through rigorous training of each one's intellectual, physical and moral qualities.

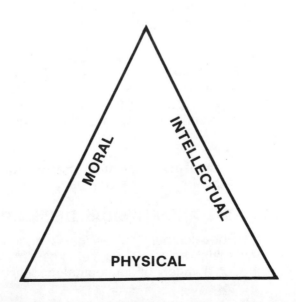

THE CONTEMPORARY PROGRAM

The contemporary approach to fitness at the Academy implies that several fundamental factors should be taken into consideration. First, individuals must be provided with correct knowledge and opportunities which enable them to train efficiently and appropriately. Secondly, the desire to continue training throughout one's lifetime must be instilled through the training.

To train effectively, the men and women of the U.S. Naval Academy Brigade are taught to understand that each component of fitness requires training principles and specific program methods. They must also realize that one's level of physical fitness is important while at the Academy, but even more so during their careers. Each must possess the ability and the desire to maintain fitness for a lifetime.

To fulfill its responsibility for each midshipman's physical development, the Naval Academy provides a broad spectrum of fitness-stimulating requirements and opportunities. The comprehensive program includes a required physical education curriculum and an intramural sports program for every midshipman. In addition, many elect to participate in the many intercollegiate sports also available at the Academy.

Physical education curriculum

In four years midshipmen are required to complete a total of 161 contact hours in this curriculum. A grade is assigned during each of the four years. This grade is based on swimming, boxing, wrestling, gymnastics, fencing and performance on physical fitness tests. Men do not participate in fencing, nor women in boxing and wrestling.

Other subjects taught to midshipmen include many of the lifetime sports such as golf, tennis, volleyball, squash, bowling and crew. Personal conditioning is emphasized along with tests in applied strength, agility, aerobic fitness and the ability to run the obstacle course.

The general purpose of the program for men and women midshipmen is spelled out in the USNA catalog:

> The program's aims are to develop skill, confidence, teamwork, endurance, agility and competitive spirit; to develop useful habits of physical fitness; to develop the capability to train and instruct others; and to develop the background and capability to withstand physical hardship. Equally important, the program aims to be enjoyable,

to provide a release from the academic routine, to develop a lasting appreciation for sports in general, and to develop individual skills in carry-over for enjoyment after graduation.

These broadly stated aims can be stated in more specific objectives as follows:

1. To develop high levels of cardiovascular fitness, muscular strength, muscular endurance and flexibility.
2. To develop qualities of personal courage, group loyalty, fair play, leadership and quick thinking while participating under pressure in highly competitive situations.
3. To develop a high degree of proficiency in aquatic skills and the confidence to meet emergency situations in the water.
4. To acquire knowledge about proper nutrition, diet and weight control as they contribute to a high level of fitness.
5. To develop skills, confidence, and the ability to defend oneself against personal attack.
6. To develop a keen interest and sufficient skill in lifetime sports to assist the individual in maintaining a high level of physical fitness after graduation.
7. To develop knowledge of the principles and methods employed in organizing, supervising and conducting athletic and physical training programs for others.

PEP Program As part of the Physical Education Curriculum, all plebes (Fourth Class men and women midshipmen) are required to participate in the PEP program. The program is a five-day-a-week (MTTFS) fitness program which begins at 6:45 A.M. as all 1400 plebes make their way to the Astroturf football field. Beginning the first week in July, the program lasts for six weeks.

The exercise programs are varied from day to day but always include elements of cardiovascular fitness, muscular strength and endurance fitness, and flexibility fitness. The circuit training method is employed in most routines to produce total fitness. In addition to the vigorous forty-five minutes of exercises, the program also incorporates competition among the companies. This competition is keen and includes seven events: Pull-ups, flexed arm hang (women), standing long jump, dips, sit-ups, Illinois Agility Run, Thomas Pentatholon and the mile run. Records are kept and points scored as part of the Academy's required intramural competition.

The PEP Program is described in greater detail in the Appendix. As exercise and fitness programs are described throughout the text, references will be made to the specific PEP routines of training.

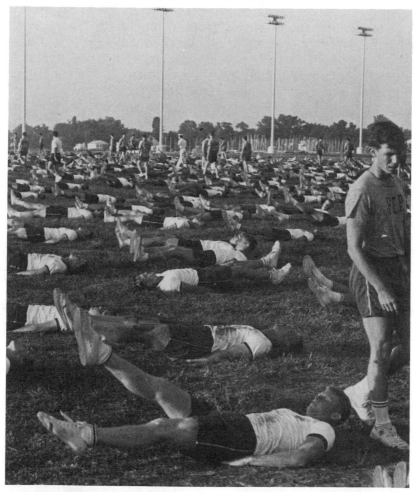

Midshipmen in the PEP Program

Physical fitness testing Another important aspect of the physical education program at the Naval Academy is measuring the fitness levels of the midshipmen. Beginning with the PEP Program in Plebe summer, all midshipmen must meet minimal fitness testing standards.

Every midshipman is tested in three areas: the mile run, applied strength and the obstacle course. The applied strength test consists of three parts: pull-ups for men; flexed arm-hang for women, standing long jump and sit-ups in two minutes. The obstacle course consists of thirteen obstacles and is 440 yards in length. Academy standards are presented in the Appendix.

Midshipmen of the United States Naval Academy are physically fit. The high degree of fitness is reflected in test results which specifically measure cardiovascular endurance, muscular strength and a combination of strength, ability, physical courage and endurance. For example, in the Spring of 1982, two hundred sixty women midshipmen established an average running time in the mile run of six (6) minutes and fifty-three (53) seconds. The results of nearly four thousand men midshipmen in the mile run when tested in 1982 indicated that the average time was 5 minutes, 47 seconds. The mode for this entire group of midshipmen was 6 min 47.5 seconds.

Twice each year all men and women midshipmen take the applied strength test. In a recent year 260 women averaged 53 seconds on the flexed-arm hang, 70.6 sit-ups in the two-minute test and 74.6 inches in the standing long jump. Both the women's results and the men's results in applied strength shown below reflect excellent levels of strength fitness.

FITNESS TEST RESULTS
OF MIDSHIPMEN AS FRESHMEN (Plebes)
Second Semesters,
Academic Years 1976-1983

TEST	Class 1980		Class 1981		Class 1982		Class 1983		Class 1984		Class 1985		Class 1986	
	WOMEN	MEN	WOMEN	MEN	WOMEN	MEN	WOMEN	MEN	WOMEN	MEN	WOMEN	MEN	WOMEN	MEN
Mile Run	7:00	5:45	7:00	5:46	6:45	5:43	6:47	5:43	6:48	5:40	6:51	5:42	6:48	5:41
Flexed-Arm Hang Pullups	23.1"	9.4	26.0"	9.5	27.8"	9.5	27.1"	10.1	28.6"	9.6	49.0"	9.8	51.9"	10.0
Standing Long Jump	—		72.9"	94.3"	73.0"	91.9"	72.9"	91.0"	74.2"	92.7"	75.3"	92.6"	74.9"	96.6"
Situps/2 minutes	60.0	72.3	65.3	72.5	68.5	71.5	65.3	71.5	63.7	71.1	69.9	71.3	67.2	71.2
Obstacle Course	3:17	2:40	3:20	2:40	3:14	2:39	3:17	2:39	3:13	2:38	3:12	2:36	3:17	2:38

TABLE 1

Personal conditioning The Naval Academy is not just interested in developing high levels of physical fitness among the midshipmen during their four years at Annapolis. Each midshipman must understand the knowledge associated with fitness and good health. The knowledge and the fitness experience will serve to motivate the future career naval officer to engage in a personal fitness program regularly throughout his or her lifetime.

The midshipman receives 12 hours of classroom instruction covering a broad range of subject matter relating to personal conditioning. The program material includes study of fundamental physical fitness principles; heart disease and fitness; stress and fitness; and nutrition (and weight management) and fitness.

Sports skills training The major focus of the Physical Education Curriculum is upon specific sports courses. The midshipman learns specific sports skills but benefits in numerous other ways from these courses. Swimming, for example, provides the midshipman with skills that can improve physical fitness, provide a relaxation or recreational outlet, and most importantly assure survival in the event of a water emergency.

Courses categorized as personal defense courses also provide opportunities to improve physical fitness but are absolutely essential to a military officer. These courses include boxing, wrestling, judo, hand-to-hand and fencing. Such combative courses additionally develop self-confidence and courage.

Other selected courses are recreationally oriented and provide excellent opportunities for lifelong fitness involvement. They include golf, tennis, handball, squash, volleyball and racquetball instruction.

Varsity and intramural athletics competition In addition to the comprehensive Physical Education Curriculum, midshipmen attending the Naval Academy are required to participate in regular intramural athletic competition and may elect to compete in the varsity sports program.

The varsity intercollegiate sports program, with 22 men's and 8 women's varsity teams, is one of the most comprehensive in the nation. The success of Navy teams is recorded in the annals of sports. Throughout the decades midshipmen have become champions in sports such as football, fencing, squash and gymnastics. Joe Bellino and Roger Staubach were Heisman Trophy winners. Twenty-seven Navy athletes have received All-American recognition. Navy heavyweight crews captured the

Olympic gold medal for eight-oared shells in Belgium in 1920, and in Finland in 1952. In the mid-60s the Navy soccer teams were undefeated in regular season competition for six years—a 48-game span. From 1960-1967, the Navy lacrosse team attained eight consecutive national championships. Captain Lloyd Keaser, USMC, a Naval Academy graduate, won the 1976 Olympic silver medal in wrestling.

In addition to the broad intercollegiate athletic program, every midshipman, with the exception of varsity athletes, must participate in the intramural sports program. The competitive sports within the Brigade of Midshipmen expand the sports opportunities and provide additional fitness and recreational opportunities.

Women may participate in all but football, fieldball, lacrosse, boxing, rugby and wrestling. Women-only sports are conducted on the battalion basis in basketball, softball, stickball and tennis. Intramural sports at the Academy include:

Basketball
Boxing
Crew
Cross-country
Fencing
Fieldball
Football
Handball
Knockabout sailing
Lacrosse
Powerlifting
Rugby
Soccer
Softball
Squash
Stickball
Swimming
Team handball
Tennis
Touch football
Track
Volleyball
Water polo
Wrestling

Women midshipmen It was only recently that the U.S. Service Academies admitted women candidates. One of the concerns was whether the women were capable of handling the intense rigors of the institutions. The following briefly describes how the women midshipmen responded at the Naval Academy.

In October 1975, President Gerald Ford signed the Defense Appropriation Authorization Act of 1976, to which an amendment had been attached directing women's admission to the service academies. This law stated that "the academic and other relevant standards required for appointment, admission, training, graduation, and commissioning of female individuals shall be the same as those required for male individuals, except for those minimum essential adjustments in such standards required because of physiological differences between male and female individuals."

The United States Naval Academy had two specific questions concerning the physical fitness training program for women. First, what were the physiological differences between men and women; and second, what were the needed adjustments in determining performance between men and women? The primary areas for concern in fitness training were muscular strength and cardiovascular endurance.

With respect to muscular strength, women on the average have somewhat less potential to build muscle tissue than men. This is primarily because biologically men have a higher percentage of lean body weight (muscle tissue) than do women. Women in turn have a higher percentage of body fat. Given the cultural tendencies to discourage women from developing muscles in their upper bodies and the natural differences in upper body strength, the pull-up test was not particularly suited to women. The Academy therefore developed the "flexed-arm hang" for women but also continued training women in pull-ups to determine the future capability of women to perform this exercise.

Men and women also differ generally in their capacities for cardiovascular endurance. Women in general have lower aerobic capacities, mainly because of smaller heart and lung capacity. This means that women must work harder aerobically to achieve the same amount of endurance work as their male companions. It has only been within the last ten to fifteen years that women were allowed and/or encouraged to participate in cardiovascular training and competitive programs.

By requiring different standards for men and women, the

Naval Academy concluded that the differences are mainly in magnitude rather than in mechanism. Women and men essentially respond to fitness training in a similar manner since the physiological and biochemical responses are the same in both sexes. Academy programs therefore accommodate both men and women equally and fairly.

THE FITNESS COMMITMENT

In this introduction we have briefly outlined the United States Naval Academy program, which is carefully designed to foster the total fitness of each midshipman. As you have discovered, the program is comprehensive, highly structured, intense and successful in reaching its objectives. Each midshipman is required to meet a high standard of physical fitness—higher than that normally demanded of civilian exercise programs.

Despite its highly structured framework, the fitness program is intensely personal for each midshipman. Each man and woman attending the Academy must accept the challenge to improve his or her level of well-being.

But how can the program presented in this book help *you* start a fitness program or improve your present fitness level? We have some sound advice which is emphasized at the Naval Academy. Study this advice and keep it in mind as you embark on your journey toward fitness and good health.

1) You must clearly understand fundamental concepts about fitness. You must understand your body and how it responds to various training methods and strategies. You must know how to proceed safely and gradually in your fitness program.

2) You must establish realistic and attainable fitness goals which correspond with your age and present level of fitness. You must above all be patient. Like good wine, the approach to the joy of fitness is a slow, gradual process.

3) Finally, your personal commitment toward improving your fitness and well-being must be strong. Fitness must become a high priority in your life and in balance with all your other desires and goals. In short, being physically fit must be prized and valued by you.

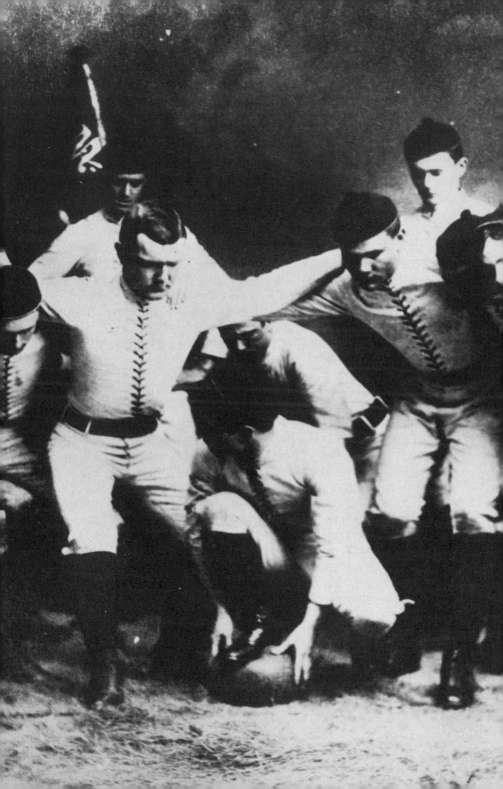

PART I
PHYSICAL FITNESS COMPONENTS

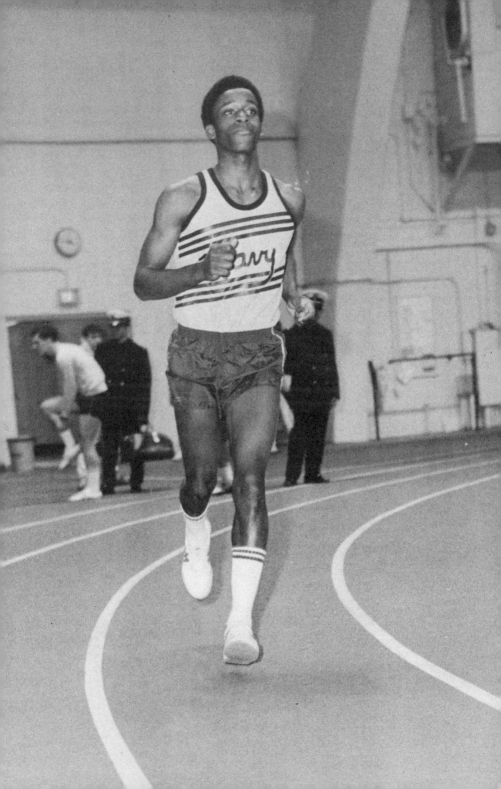

UNDERSTANDING PHYSICAL FITNESS

Physical fitness is not only one of the most important keys to a healthy body, it is the basis of dynamic and creative intellectual activity.... Intelligence and skill can only function at the peak of their capacity when the body is healthy and strong.

—President John F. Kennedy

OBJECTIVES

- Define each of the three health-related components of physical fitness.

- Identify the six skill-related components of fitness.

- Explain how one goes about achieving total fitness.

- Describe three pre-fitness program considerations.

- List three important factors to consider when setting physical fitness goals and objectives.

- Discuss the component phases of a typical exercise or conditioning program routine.

DEFINING PHYSICAL FITNESS

Physical fitness for some individuals means having a high level of skill proficiency in a sport. Others might view physical fitness as having an attractive physical shape. The popular emphasis upon body building for men and women leads many to believe that physical fitness and a well-proportioned body are directly interrelated. We often think of persons with a neat appearance and an alert demeanor as representing the fitness model.

These and other subjective descriptions of being "in shape" often reflect opinions about self-image, and sometimes are misleading. A clearer definition of physical fitness requires an observation of the functional considerations of physical performance. Perhaps the simplest definition of physical fitness is "the capacity of an individual to perform sustained physical effort."

Of course this definition requires further clarification. What is meant by "sustained physical effort?" What anatomical and physiological factors enable one to sustain this effort, and how does one improve one's capacity to sustain physical effort? First let us examine what most exercise professionals consider to be the most essential components of physical fitness.

COMPONENTS OF PHYSICAL FITNESS

Exercise specialists often separate the components of physical fitness into health-related and skill-related components.[1] The development of skill-related components is essential to the improvement of athletic skills and is indirectly related to physical fitness. Because the more general health-related components have direct application to the development of physical fitness at all age levels, our primary focus in this text will be upon these components.

HEALTH-RELATED COMPONENTS[2]

Within the scope of this text, physical fitness will be described as having three major health-related components. These include: 1) cardiovascular (aerobics) fitness, 2) muscular fitness (comprising muscular strength and muscular endurance) and 3) flexiblity fitness.

Some fitness experts include body composition (the extent of an individual's body fat-leanness ratio) as an additional health-related component. We prefer to treat this important aspect of health fitness as a separate and comprehensive unit under nutrition and weight control.

Cardiovascular fitness The ability of the heart, lungs and circulatory system to sustain exercise for long periods of time is defined as cardiovascular fitness. Terms such as aerobics, cardiorespiratory, and cardiopulmonary essentially mean the same as cardiovascular when used in the exercise context. Dr. Kenneth Cooper's popular aerobics programs are all geared toward the improvement of cardiovascular fitness. Aerobics refers to the body's efficiency with which it can utilize oxygen or air—thus providing an ideal way to measure one's cardiovascular fitness.

Muscular fitness Consists of two elements (muscular strength and muscular endurance). Muscular fitness is defined as the ability of skeletal muscles to exert maximum force (muscular strength) and to sustain repeated muscular effort (muscular endurance).

Flexibility fitness The third component of physical fitness, flexibility fitness, is defined as the ability to achieve full range of movement at the various joints of the body. Specifically, it refers to the ability of the soft connective tissue (muscle, fascia, tendons and ligaments) to stretch during movement.

SKILL-RELATED COMPONENTS

These components are essential to the development and maintenance of sports and athletic skills. Through appropriate practice, these components can greatly improve such skills. They are also important to consider in instances where an individual cannot perform fitness-promoting activities. Correction of these deficiencies will obviously assist such individuals improve fitness.

Since detailed discussions of the skill-related components are more appropriate to specific sports skills books and kinesiological or exercise physiology texts, we will limit our emphasis to the definitions only.[3]

- Agility: the ability to change the position of your body quickly and to control the movement of your whole body.
- Balance: the ability to keep an upright posture while you are standing still or moving.
- Coordination: the ability to use your senses, such as your eyes, together with your body parts, such as your arms, or to use two or more body parts together.
- Power: the ability to do strength performances quickly. Power involves both strength and speed.
- Reaction Time: the amount of time it takes you to get moving once you see the need to move.
- Speed: the ability to perform a movement or cover a distance in a short period of time.

Note: Sharkey[4] includes flexibility fitness as another element of muscular fitness.

ACHIEVING TOTAL FITNESS

The programs at the U.S. Naval Academy are designed to enhance both the skill- and health-related fitness components of each midshipman. Total fitness (or high-level wellness) is represented and achieved through proper exercise, good nutrition, managing weight, controlling stress and appropriate rest and relaxation. An attitude of preventive health maintenance is an additional contributing factor in the health of all midshipmen.

These factors are not only regarded as important for each Brigade member, but they are considered *essential* for each future naval officer.

Through a highly competitive intramural and varsity sports program, a comprehensive physical activity curriculum, and a rigorous fitness program all health- and skill-related components of fitness are optimally developed. The U.S. Naval Academy has traditionally emphasized total fitness and will continue to do so because of the excellent quality achieved in its officers.

PRE-PHYSICAL FITNESS PROGRAM
CONSIDERATION

Regardless of your sex or age, there are three essential factors which merit consideration prior to starting an exercise program.

Medical evaluation A regular medical examination is essential to detect early signs of illness and disease, especially as we grow older. The aging process makes us more susceptible to certain degenerative illnesses. Periodic medical evaluations are therefore important health care measures.

These evaluations are even more important if we decide to initiate an exercise program after a few years of inactivity. Because we generally become more sedentary as we age, it is wise for anyone over thirty-five and all others who are seriously deconditioned to obtain a medical assessment prior to starting vigorous or strenuous exercise.

In addition to the medical evaluation, some physicians recommend an exercise stress (tolerance) test before starting a program.[5] Persons with known heart disease risk factors regardless of age should also consult their physician about a pre-screening exercise ECG test. This group may include persons who smoke heavily, are obese, have high blood pressure, are diabetic, or have a family history of heart disease. In general, a thorough medical evaluation includes a comprehensive medical history, a detailed physical examination, and blood and other laboratory tests where appropriate.

Your desired exercise program should be discussed thoroughly with your physician, and any prescribed limitations and/or exercise restrictions followed until otherwise noted.

Present level fitness evaluation Many individuals begin exercising safely without extensive medical testing. Although a pre-program fitness evaluation is not always necessary if one starts very slowly and progresses cautiously in a desirable and appropriate program, remember that most exercise injuries are experienced early in one's conditioning program. Many of us attempt to speed up our conditioning efforts. Overexertion early in a program can lead to joint and muscle stress which could abruptly halt a well-designed program.

Some individuals are interested to know approximately how fit they are before starting a program. This information will help them set more realistic goals for themselves. If you desire to know your pre-program fitness level, several options are available to you.

1) One option is to find a center in your geographic area that performs submaximal treadmill tests of fitness. Generally this test

measures the cardiovascular fitness level by having you exercise to a safe point of fatigue, usually not exceeding eighty-five percent of your maximal effort. Your maximum capacity for exercise is then predicted based upon these results. Your blood pressure and ECG are monitored throughout the treadmill or bicycle test. Check local community colleges, YMCAs and hospitals or health centers in your area to determine if they offer such services. Usually there is a moderate fee for the testing service.

2) Another option for the non-obese young healthy adult (18-35 years) is the Cooper Aerobics Fitness Test.[6] Cooper describes these tests in detail and offers a 12-minute run/walk, a 12-minute cycle, a 12-minute swimming, a 1.5 mile run/walk, and a 3.0 mile walk as options. Cooper does not personally recommend the tests until an individual has trained at least six weeks on one of his aerobic starter programs. Certainly it is advisable not to do the test without several weeks of gradual preparation.

In addition, when you decide to take an aerobics test, do not exert yourself over eighty-five percent of maximal heart rate. After several months of gradual conditioning, there will be ample time to periodically self-administer the test.

Self-appraisal of fitness readiness In addition to the medical evaluation and the pre-fitness evaluation, you may wish to do a broadly-based self-appraisal to determine your readiness for a conditioning program. Answer the following questions honestly and discuss the answers with a fitness specialist to help you plan a program which is compatible with your readiness evaluation.

- How long has it been since you participated in a regular conditioning program? What type of a program was it?
- Are you carrying more than 25 percent body fat? How recently did you gain the weight that increased your fat level to this point?
- Are you under personal stress which you feel you are not able to control effectively?
- Do you use medications or substances which alter your normal physiological state and could make certain exercise inappropriate for you?
- Do you have any serious medical problems or recent injuries which might require certain exercise restrictions?

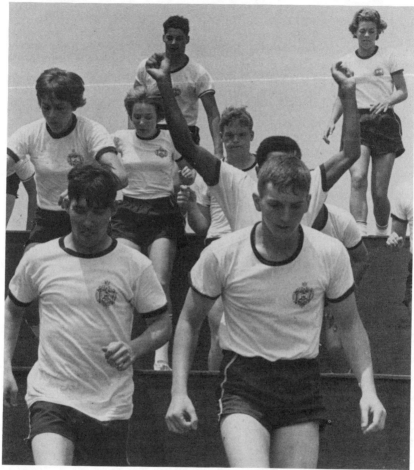

Fitness means overcoming obstacles and meeting challenges.

PHYSICAL FITNESS GOALS AND OBJECTIVES

Following a thorough pre-assessment of your readiness for an exercise program, you should carefully plan short-term objectives and long-range goals. You may wish to discuss these plans with an exercise specialist, your physician or someone who has experienced a gradually progressive fitness program.

Minimally, your goals and objectives should take into consideration the development of all three fitness elements (cardiovascular, muscular and flexibility fitness). You may also wish to include broader behavior changes in stress management, weight control and nutrition.

Write your goals and objectives down. When placed in writing they will serve as a powerful motivator for you and assure you that you are following a safe and progressive program.

If possible, you may want to enroll in a supervised fitness class instead of setting out on your own. Most American communities offer these courses at public schools in the evening, at community colleges, at local YMCAs and at various private centers. Be sure you have a well-qualified or certified instructor.

Realistic goals and objectives Your goals and objectives must be designed within your ability range. Many deconditioned individuals returning to an exercise program expect immediate results and proceed too fast.

These attitudes and attempts often result in personal injury, severe muscular and joint soreness, and subsequent withdrawal from the program. Realistic goals and objectives should follow the old adage "train, do not strain." In short this means progessing slowly and safely. Allow exercise to become a joyful pleasure rather than routine drudgery.

Motivation "Getting psyched" about your exercise program and finding motivational aids to keep you going are important considerations. Few individuals have the self-discipline to initiate and continue a regular exercise program without adequate motivation.

Motivators may take the form of a good friend who willingly agrees to participate with you. Oftentimes each of you will serve as a motivator for the other, particularly on those "low energy" days.

You might also become motivated because you desire to compete in a sport which requires an improved level of fitness. People who take up skiing, for example, know that the sport requires leg strength, endurance and coordination—factors which assure safe participation and are developed in a conditioning program.

The desire to feel better about yourself or to fit into your bathing suit or your new clothes is also a strong exercise motivator. For many others a powerful motivator is improved health, both mental and physical.

Regardless of your initial motivator, remember that everyone may have different reasons for starting an exercise program and may find that their reasons for continuing a program change periodically. If you desire to start a program and cannot think of why you want to do it, good advice is not to worry about the reason. You will think of plenty of reasons after you experience fitness.

Monitoring your progress Many individuals discover that a journal or personal diary is very helpful in measuring progress. Fitness milestones of progress can be noted (and rewarded), pleasure can be gained from noting these achievements, and the impetus to reach new levels of personal fitness results from keeping a personal journal.

Record keeping is not essential, however, and many exercisers find the chore tedious. But if you are the type of person who finds it difficult to stay on an exercise schedule, a diary may help. When your program becomes routine and a regular part of your lifestyle you may wish to discard the journal-keeping chore.

EXERCISE CONDITIONING ROUTINE

As mentioned often throughout this book, the two paramount concerns are that you exercise *safely* and progress *slowly*, regardless of the routine you follow. Cardiovascular, muscular and flexibility fitness programs demand patience on your part. Exercise is the stimulus which causes adaptations or changes in the way your body functions. Physiological and anatomical changes require time and cannot be rushed.

Most exercise specialists agree that a general physical fitness program should include 1) a warmup, 2) a main routine incorporating elements of aerobic, anaerobic and flexibility training, and 3) a cool-down.

Competing athletes must also include specific practice of the many skill-related components of fitness as well. For those of you who prefer to use participation in a vigorous sport as your regular exercise, be sure to include a warmup and a cool-down as part of your program.

Warmup Every exercise, conditioning or sports session should be preceded by a warmup. One purpose of warming up is to prevent injury by stretching (elongating) the muscles that you intend to use during your exercise period. The warmup, which generally includes static stretching, as well as slow isotonic movements at full range of mobility, is also designed to raise the muscle temperature several degrees. This is an added precautionary measure to prevent injury.

These slow static, rhythmical movements slowly increase the heart rate. When they are followed by large muscle calisthenics, they gradually raise the heart rate to training levels. During this 5-15 minute warmup session which focuses on flexibility and on gradually increasing heart rate, you should be at the lower level of your *training zone* (50-70% of your maximum capacity).

Main exercise segment Ideally, exercises to promote general well-being and fitness should contain cardiovascular (aerobic) and muscular (anaerobic) components. If your program contains a flexibility component, you get a bonus.

To assure total fitness, many individuals include an aerobic (running, jogging, walking, swimming, cycling) phase with an anaerobic (weight training, heavy calisthenics) phase. Perhaps because of the recent interest in triathlons and multi-sport participation by many individuals, there has been a renewed interest in circuit training. This total development program will be discussed in a later chapter.

How you arrange the various components of your exercise routine depends somewhat upon your desired outcomes. You may wish to emphasize your aerobic component over your anaerobic component or vice versa. Benefits from each component result only, however, if you follow certain principles of training such as intensity, duration and frequency. These will be discussed in detail in the respective chapters on each component of fitness.

If you elect to develop and maintain your physical fitness through active participation in individual, dual or team sports, a separate chapter has been written to understand the benefits and limitations of these activities.

Cool-down Following vigorous exercise, it is very important to ease your heart rate down to lower levels. This should never be done by immediately remaining immobile (lying or sitting) following exercise. A slow jog, walk, mild calisthenics or stretching are recommended until your heart rate falls at least below your lower level training zone.

Various authors recommend that your heart rate drop below a specific figure before you shower. A more realistic measure is that it should fall to within 20-30 beats of resting rate within five to ten minutes after exercise. The severity of the exercise and environment (temperature and humidity) will affect how rapidly your heart rate recovers and how low it will go immediately following exercise. However, do not expect it to drop to resting levels.

REFERENCES

1. Corbin, Charles B. and Ruth Lindsey, *The Ultimate Fitness Book.* New York, NY: Leisure Press, 1984.
2. ibid., pp. 12.
3. ibid., pp. 10.
4. Sharkey, Brian, *Physiology of Fitness.* Champaign, IL: Human Kinetics Publishers, 1979, p. 4.
5. Cooper, Kenneth H. *The Aerobics Way.* New York, NY: Bantam Books (paperback), 1978, p. 52.
6. ibid., pp. 87-92.
7. Note: The term "training zone" refers to an exercise heart rate level required to produce a cardiovascular training effect. It will be explained in Chapter 2.

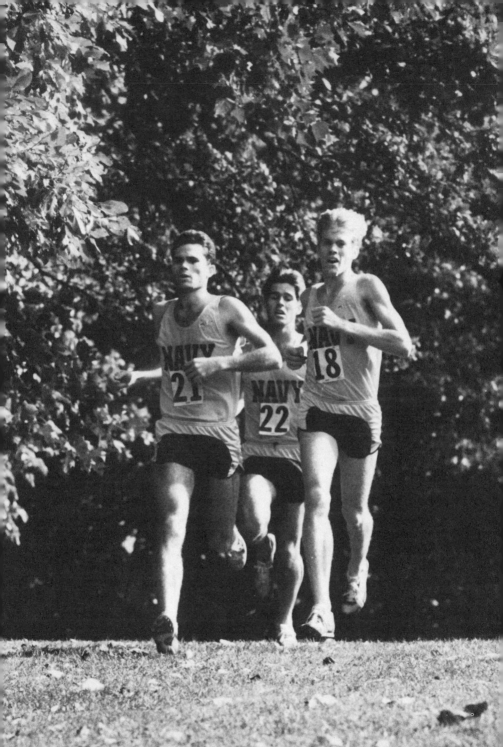

CARDIOVASCULAR FITNESS —AEROBICS

We have long been the richest nation in the world; now let's be the healthiest. That is not a matter of curing diseases, but preventing them. Exercise is a major factor in disease prevention. Those who exercise even enjoy sex more, and if that isn't a motivating factor, I don't know what is!

Jesse Steinfeld, M.D.
Past Surgeon General

OBJECTIVES

- Define the term "cardiovascular fitness" and explain the principles for achieving it.
- Discuss the frequency, duration and intensity principles of aerobic training.
- Describe other training procedures and how they are important.
- Define and discuss aerobic and anaerobic training and the Cooper aerobics point system.
- Present specific programs in jogging, swimming, continuous rhythmic exercises and cycling.
- Identify results and benefits achieved through cardiovascular and aerobic fitness training.

Chapter 2 emphasizes how serious a threat cardiovascular disease has become to our nation—documentation now shows it to be the leading cause of death among all degenerative diseases. But evidence continues to mount that appropriate types of physical activities may prevent cardiovascular disease—prevention, rather than cure, is indeed the key.

CARDIOVASCULAR (AEROBIC) FITNESS

Cardiovascular fitness

The term is easily understood—it is simply an indication of the individual's ability to take in and process large amounts of oxygen to enable the body to maintain periods of extended physical activity without diminished efficiency.

Aerobic fitness

The well-known sports medicine physician Dr. Kenneth H. Cooper has redefined the term "cardiovascular fitness" by including the concept of aerobics. To train aerobically means to train with oxygen. The capability to take in and process oxygen is a significant factor in cardiovascular fitness, and an excellent indication of your personal cardiovascular fitness is the number of liters of oxygen you can process each minute. After you have trained for at least six weeks, you may wish to try the Three Minute Step Test, on page 48, to obtain information regarding your oxygen capability.

Heart rate and aerobic fitness

Heart rate, the number of times the heart beats each minute, is indeed the key to aerobic fitness. It is easy to check—simply count the number of times your pulse beats in a minute. The count may be taken at the wrist or at the carotid artery, as illustrated in Figures 1 and 2 following.

A sweep second hand on a wristwatch may be used to time the count. Count your pulse with the index and middle fingers, not with your thumb—that would give you a faulty count.

Understanding heart rates

Resting heart rate (RHR) The resting heart rate is to be established upon first awakening in the morning. Count the pulse for 60 seconds before rising. Do this on three different mornings and use the average of three counts. *The higher the degree of fitness, the lower the resting heart rate.* The average of the brigade's resting heart rates (RHR) is 66 beats/min.

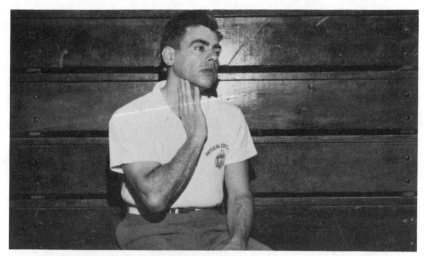

Figure 1: Pulse count at carotid artery

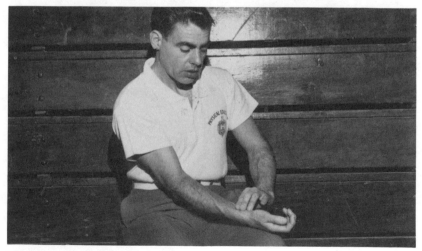

Figure 2: Pulse count at wrist

Working heart rate (WHR) The working rate can be established during any chosen exercises of any nature. During any training routine, stop, and instantly count the pulse rate for ten seconds. Multiply by six. This establishes the working heart rate for one minute. Obviously, it is necessary to have a stopwatch or a sweep second hand on a wristwatch.

Maximum heart rate (MHR) When an individual pushes himself to *maximum* capability in any endurance event, then stops and instantly takes his heart rate for 10 seconds, he establishes his maximum heart rate (MHR). According to one physiologist, the subject runs a half-mile as rapidly as his condition permits. Then, at the end, the pulse is instantly counted for ten seconds and multiplied by six. It should be understood, however, that such a procedure is applicable only if the individual is not over 35 years of age and is in a highly trained state. At the Naval Academy all entering midshipmen establish their maximum heart rate in the described manner.

For most of those desiring to establish their maximum heart rate, a simple method of calculation can be used. The number 220 is assumed to be the base number. From that number, it is simply a question of subtracting one's age. For example, if an individual is 30 years of age, the maximum heart rate is estimated as follows: 220 - 30 = 190 estimated beats per minute, under maximum stress conditions.

THREE MAJOR PRINCIPLES OF AEROBIC TRAINING

There are three major training principles to be observed if the selected training program is to contribute to an adequate degree of cardiovascular fitness.

These three principles[1] depend on the frequency, duration and intensity of the selected activity. The requirements for these principles are as follows:

> FREQUENCY Train three to four times per week
> DURATION Train 15-60 minutes each session*
> INTENSITY Train at or above the required working heart rate

The frequency and duration principles are readily understood. The intensity principle, however, which requires a training zone, or an appropriate range of the required working heart rate, needs to be examined in detail.

Training intensity guides
At the Naval Academy midshipmen are taught to establish their working heart rate as follows: To establish the required training

*At USNA 35 minutes is the minimum

rate for cardiovascular fitness, the following formula is used. Subtract the subject's resting heart rate from the subject's maximum heart rate. Calculate 75% of the difference. To that result add the subject's resting heart rate. Thus, if a midshipman has as heart rates MHR = 200 beats per minute and RHR = 60 bpm, his required working heart rate would be calculated as follows: 200 - 60 = 140; 75% of 140 = 105; add 60, and the result is 165 bpm— the number of beats required by this midshipman if he is to achieve a training effect for cardiovascular fitness.

Formula WHR = .75 (MHR - RHR) + RHR (according to M.J. Karvonen, as described by H.A. DeVries)[2]

It has been determined that those midshipmen who are in fair to good condition should take 75% to establish their required working heart rate. Those who wish to attain a higher level of cardiovascular fitness may use as much as 85-90% to establish their heart rate.

More specific information is included as a guide to determine the appropriate training intensity. It is desirable for each individual to determine the actual range of the number of times each minute the heart should beat while training. By referring to Table 1 it is possible to determine that range by calculating the appropriate training zone. For example, let us assume that an individual is 35 years of age and in less than satisfactory condition. To establish the required intensity, it will be necessary to determine his training zone.

Again, using the same formula, but with a 65% base, WHR = 65% (MHR - RHR) + RHR, we determine the required working heart rate as follows:

> MHR: Age of the individual is 35; thus, 220 - 35 = 185
> RHR: Established by pulse count: 72 beats per minute
> *Calculation*: 185 - 72 = 113; 65% of 113 = 73.5; add 72, the resting heart rate, to that (73.5 + 72), and the result is 145.5 or 146 beats per minute. As is indicated in Table 1, the training zone ranges from 140 beats per minute to 151 beats per minute.

TRAINING INTENSITY GUIDE
(BASED UPON AVERAGE RESTING HR OF 72)

AGE	MAX HR PER MIN.	TRAINING HEART RATE ZONES		
		60-70% Poor-Fair Condition & (Heart Patients)	70-80% Fair-Good Condition	80-90% Good-Excellent Condition
—20	200	(25) 149—162	(27) 162—174	(29) 174—187
—25	195	(24) 146—158	(26) 158—170	(28) 170—183
—30	190	(23) 143—155	(26) 155—166	(28) 166—179
—35	185	(23) 140—151	(25) 151—162	(27) 162—176
—40	180	(23) 137—148	(25) 148—158	(27) 158—171
—45	175	(22) 134—144	(24) 144—154	(26) 154—168
—50	170	(21) 131—141	(24) 141—150	(25) 150—164
—55	165	(21) 128—137	(23) 137—146	(24) 146—161
—60	160	(21) 125—134	(23) 134—142	(24) 142—157

TO CALCULATE YOUR ACTUAL TRAINING ZONE:
TRAINING ZONE = (MAX HR-RESTING HR) × % + RESTING HR
LEVEL DESIRED

TABLE 2

ADDITIONAL TRAINING PRECEDURES

Warmup

It is extremely important to spend time in preparing your body for a training session. This aspect of training is frequently ignored and results in unnecessary and frustrating injuries such as painful muscle pulls or strains. The purpose of warming up is to stretch muscles of the back, arms and legs and also to increase the working heart rate so that your circulatory system can slowly be prepared for the higher heart rate as an increasing number of liters of oxygen are required by the body. Midshipmen are encouraged to warm up and to saturate their muscles with blood to prevent unnecessary injuries. They are encouraged to carry out three to five minutes of exercises of an easy nature, such as jumping, bending, stretching and gentle twisting.

The Warmup Do the following exercises, sixty seconds each.

1. The Side-straddle Hop
2. Bending and Twisting
3. Crawl Stroke Forward
4. Crawl Stroke Backward
5. Butterfly

Note: Exercises are pictured in this chapter under Cardiovascular Routine, Program #2.

The side-straddle hop is often called the jumping jack. A lot of springing action is encouraged; arms should be straight, open hands touching over the head.

In the bending and twisting exercise, the lead arm should be straight, and the trading arm angled. We encourage a lot of ankle, hip and shoulder action.

The butterfly is named after the swimmer's butterfly stroke. Both arms complete a circle. As the arms are extended behind the body, shoulders are lifted and arms and hands are extended over the head.

Breathing

The key is to bring oxygen into your body. You need remember only that natural breathing is always correct. Always avoid breath-holding. It is desirable to breathe as fully and deeply as possible. Deep ventilation wards off fatigue.

Overload (gradual increase of intensity)

As indicated in Table 1, in the Training Intensity Guide, individuals in an untrained state begin at a low level of intensity. It is recommended that the working heart rate be established by applying the 60%-70% base. Research has shown that a time period of six weeks is required before any cardiovascular foundation can be established. After six weeks the intensity may be increased, depending on the training goals of the individual. When examining the suggested training exercises and programs in this chapter, it will be noted that not all days are of equal intensity. On certain days a greater intensity is suggested than on others. Your body requires a definite resting phase after every hard training day. As a rule, hard training days should be alternated with easier training days. It must be understood, however, that cardiovascular fitness levels cannot improve unless increasingly greater demands are periodically made of the heart and lungs. How frequently the intensity is increased, and to what extent, is determined by the level of physical fitness the individual hopes to achieve. The rule is that progression should come slowly and with small increments.

Recuperation rule

After you have trained at the appropriate working heart rate for 35 or 40 minutes, keep moving. Don't sit down. If you walk slowly, your body will recover more quickly. The reason you are fatigued at the end of a demanding cardiovascular workout is that you have reached your oxygen intake capability. Your body was unable to take in the required number of liters, and it reached a state called "oxygen debt." As you slow down, you feel better, because you begin to repay your oxygen debt. It is a physiological fact that you recover more quickly and efficiently if you walk around leisurely. It is definitely harmful to extend one's body and suddenly stop all physical activity, rather than to slow down gradually for another five to ten minutes.

Time of workout

Most people find that they train best 3-4 hours after a meal. Many train before breakfast, some during the noon hour, others in the evening, after their work day. It is possible to adapt to any reasonable schedule. The hour of training is set by the individual, depending on work responsibilities and personal preference.

Anaerobic and aerobic training methods

Anaerobic training will achieve a distinct level of physical fitness. However, the cardiovascular system is not necessarily trained. Anaerobic exercise implies training without making oxygen demands on the cardiovascular system. Two types of activities come to mind. First, underwater swimming is strictly an anaerobic exercise. Sprinting is another anaerobic exercise. A sprinter may be the winner of the gold medal in the Olympic Games, yet not have adequate endurance to demonstrate a minimum degree of cardiovascular fitness. Dr. Kenneth Cooper demonstrated this fact with Hasely Crawford of Trinidad, a gold medal winner in 1976. When tested in cardiovascular fitness, he was able to continue the exercise for only 16½ minutes, which would classify this world class sprinter as "poor" in cardiovascular fitness. This is not difficult to understand if one considers that the champion's training was exclusively in sprints and with weights, but not in cardiovascular endurance.

When Dr. Cooper visited the Naval Academy in 1972, he explained how a maximum training effect was achieved through maximum aerobic participation. He illustrated his point as follows:

	AEROBIC IMPACT IN PERCENT	ANAEROBIC IMPACT IN PERCENT
100-yard run	1%	99%
The marathon	95%	5%
The mile run	55%	45%
The 1½-mile run	85%	15%

It is of interest to note that the mile and a half has a significantly greater impact aerobically than the mile run. It is better to slow down a bit and to run the mile and a half than to run a very fast mile.

DETERMINING YOUR LEVEL
OF CARDIOVASCULAR FITNESS

Now that you have become familiar with the three major aerobic training principles and additional training factors, you need to determine your state of health and your level of cardiovascular fitness. Then you will be prepared to begin that training program most suited to your health, personal desires and age. Remember, before you begin to train it is recommended that you consult your physician. Let us now assume that you have consulted your physician and he has determined that you may begin a moderate cardiovascular training program.

The training intensity guide will tell you how hard you should train. You will probably wish to find out how fit you are at this point. If you are certain that you are in the poor to fair category, you may use the appropriate column in the Training Guide on page 42. If you have already trained appropriately for at least six to eight weeks, you may wish to evaluate your level of aerobic capacity by taking the Three-Minute Step Test or one of Cooper's Twelve-Minute Tests.

The three tests are described in detail on the following pages. You will note that only one of these tests, the 60-Second Test, is recommended if you are in a deconditioned state. Just because an individual at one time had achieved a distinctly high level of aerobic fitness does not make it possible for him or her to begin training at that level achieved six months, a year or ten years in the past. Physical fitness training cannot be considered a deposit in the bank. The initial level is lost unless regular deposits continue to be made at least three or four times every week.

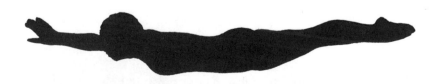

The 60-Second Step Test:

- PARTICIPANTS: Anyone declared by a physician healthy enough to begin a cardiovascular training program.

- LENGTH: 60 seconds.

- INTENSITY: 30 steps for the 60 seconds.

- RECOVERY: Pulse count begins 30 seconds after exercise is stopped. Take pulse count for 30 seconds.

- HOW TO TEST: Consult the Three-Minute Step Test on pages 48-50.

- YOUR SCORE: Consult the Scoring Table below. Enter your scores below in RECORDS.

Scoring Table

YOUR CATEGORY	30-Second Count PULSE BEATS
Good	30 - 47 beats
Average	48 - 64 beats
Poor	65 - 80 beats

SIXTY-SECOND STEP TEST RECORDS

	First Test	After 3 weeks	After 6 weeks
Date			
30-second count			
Your category (see above)			

- COMMENTS: After six weeks participants will probably wish to evaluate their fitness by taking the Three-Minute Test. Scores for this test were developed from an Adult Physical Fitness Program administered to faculty and staff at the United States Naval Academy.

The Three-Minute Step Test

- PARTICIPANTS: Anyone declared by a physician to be healthy enough to train cardiovascularly, and those participants who have trained regularly for six weeks, three times a week, at the appropriate level of intensity.

- LENGTH: Three minutes.

- INTENSITY: Men: Step at the rate of 24 steps per minute.
  Women: Step at the rate of 22 steps per minute.

- STEPPING SURFACE: Should be 16¼" high. If a chair is used, the scores will not be entirely accurate; since a chair is slightly higher, the test would be more difficult.

- RECOVERY: Pulse count begins five seconds after exercise is stopped. Remain standing. After five seconds count your pulse for 15 seconds and multiply by four.

- YOUR SCORE: Consult the Scoring Table on page 50. Note that your score will give you your oxygen capability; the closer you rank to the 100th percentile, the better you are. Enter your score in "Records" on page 50.

- HOW YOU DO IT:
  1. Place your right foot on surface to prepare for test.
  2. Start 3-minute count.
  3. Bring your left foot up on surface.
  4. Step down with your right foot.
  5. Step down with your left foot.
  6. Bring your right foot up on surface.
  7. Continue: up, up, down, down.

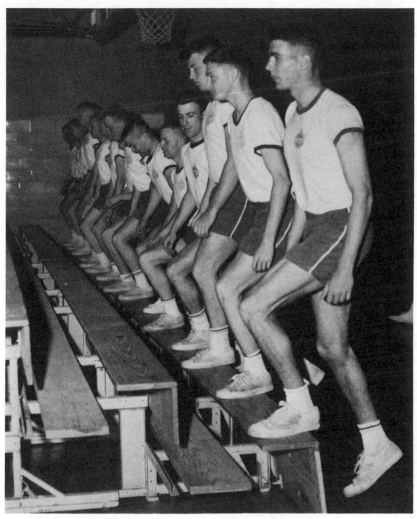

First class midshipmen perform Three-Minute Step Test

THE THREE-MINUTE STEP TEST - SCORING TABLES
(for Men and Women of College Age)

PERCENTILE RANKING	RECOVERY HR FEMALE	PREDICTED MAX VO2a (ml/kg min)	RECOVERY HR MALE	PREDICTED MAX VO2 (ml/kg min)
100	128	42.2	120	60.9
95	140	40.0	124	59.3
90	148	38.5	128	57.6
85	152	37.7	136	54.2
80	156	37.0	140	52.5
75	158	36.6	144	50.9
70	160	36.3	148	49.2
65	162	35.9	149	48.8
60	163	35.7	152	47.5
55	164	35.5	154	46.7
50	166	35.1	156	45.8
45	168	34.8	160	44.1
40	170	34.4	162	43.3
35	171	34.2	164	42.5
30	172	34.0	166	41.6
25	176	33.3	168	40.8
20	180	32.6	172	39.1
15	182	32.2	176	37.4
10	184	31.8	178	36.6
5	196	29.6	184	34.1

From F. Katch and W. McArdie, *Nutrition, Weight Control and Exercise,* Boston, Houghton-Mifflin Co., 1977.

RECORDS

	First Month	Second Month	Third Month	AVERAGE
Score 60 sec.				
DATE	5th	6th	7th	
Score 60 sec.				
DATE	9th	10th	11th	
Score 60 sec.				
DATE				

COMMENTS: If the test is carried out precisely as previously described, it is possible to establish oxygen capability and percentile ranking. For those who wish to do so, it is recommended that a metronome be used.

However, it is also possible to change the intensity to 30 steps per minute and to use a chair for stepping. In this case, the test is of great value if it is taken periodically and the individual keeps track of scores and continues to compare later scores with scores achieved earlier. It is highly motivating to continue to train aerobically as one observes that the recovery pulse rate decreases.

Cooper's Twelve-Minute Tests

Before the twelve-minute tests are considered, it is desirable to understand a little more about Dr. Cooper's aerobics program. Cooper measured the amount of oxygen consumed by men and women of all ages during exercise. Oxygen consumption is measured in milliliters per kilogram of total body weight per minute. Such a measurement tells the researcher basically how much oxygen the body is consuming, canceling out differences resulting from variation in body weight. Dr. Cooper measured individual oxygen consumption in a large variety of endurance events. He translated the milliliter figures into exercise points, then determined that the average citizen would be required to earn 27 points (women) 35 points (men) each week. This internationally renowned sports medicine physician then developed a point system for many different types of physical activity. From his research Cooper knew precisely how far and how fast an individual had to run to demonstrate varying degrees of cardiovascular fitness. Accordingly he developed a twelve-minute running test for men and women to evaluate aerobic fitness. The test follows.

THE POINT SYSTEM
Walking/Running

Time (hr:min:sec) 1.0 Mile	Point Value
Over 20:01	0
20:00-15:01	1.0
15:00-12:01	2.0
12:00-10:01	3.0
10:00- 8:01	4.0
8:00- 6:41	5.0
6:40- 5:44	6.0
under 5:43	7.0

It must be understood that those who choose to test their fitness level should have an adequate level of aerobic fitness. It is recommended that this test not be attempted unless individuals have already trained for a period of at least six weeks, at the appropriate intensity, as discussed earlier.

Another means of evaluating one's aerobic fitness is the 1.5-mile run test illustrated on page 53. It may be easier to run a distance which is measured than to run a certain length of time and then evaluate the distance covered. It is obvious that this test, similar to Cooper's 12-minute test, requires a distinctly adequate level of training before it is attempted.

12-Minute Walking/Running Test
Distance (Miles) Covered in 12 Minutes

Fitness Category		13-19	20-29	30-39	40-49	50-59	60+
				Age (years)			
I. Very Poor	(men)	<1.30*	<1.22	<1.18	<1.14	<1.03	<.87
	(women)	<1.0	<.96	<.94	<.88	<.84	<.78
II. Poor	(men)	1.30-1.37	1.22-1.31	1.18-1.30	1.14-1.24	1.03-1.16	.87-1.02
	(women)	1.00-1.18	.96-1.11	95.105	.88-.98	.84-.93	.78-.86
III. Fair	(men)	1.38-1.56	1.32-1.49	1.31-1.45	1.25-1.39	1.17-1.30	1.03-1.20
	(women)	1.19-1.29	1.12-1.22	1.06-1.18	.99-1.11	.94-1.05	.87-.98
IV. Good	(men)	1.57-1.72	1.50-1.64	1.46-1.56	1.40-1.53	1.31-1.44	1.21-1.32
	(women)	1.30-1.43	1.23-1.34	1.19-1.29	1.12-1.24	1.06-1.18	.99-1.09
V. Excellent	(men)	1.73-1.86	1.65-1.76	1.57-1.69	1.54-1.65	1.45-1.58	1.33-155
	(women)	1.44-1.51	1.35-1.45	1.30-1.39	1.25-1.34	1.19-1.30	1.10-1.18
VI. Superior	(men)	>1.87	>1.77	>1.70	>1.66	>1.59	>1.56
	(women)	>1.52	>1.46	>1.40	>1.35	>1.31	>1.19

*< Means "less than"; > means "more than."

1.5-MILE RUN TEST
Time (Minutes)
Age (years)

Fitness Category		13-19	20-29	30-39	40-49	50-59	60+
I. Very poor	(men)	<15:31*	<16:01	<16:31	<17:31	<19:01	<20:01
	(women)	<18:31	<19:01	<19:31	<20:01	<20:31	<21:01
II. Poor	(men)	12:11-15:30	14:01-16:00	14:44-16:30	15:36-17:30	17:01-19:00	19:01-20:00
	(women)	16:55-18:30	18:31-19:00	19:01-19:30	19:31-20:00	20:01-20:30	21:00-21:31
III. Fair	(men)	10:49-12:10	12:01-14:00	12:31-14:45	13:01-15:35	14:31-17:00	16:16-19:00
	(women)	14:31-16:54	15:55-18:30	16:31-19:00	17:31-19:30	19:01-20:00	19:31-20:30
IV. Good	(men)	9:41-10:48	10:46-12:00	11:01-12:30	11:31-13:00	12:31-14:30	14:00-16:15
	(women)	12:30-14:30	13:31-15:54	14:31-16:30	15:56-17:30	16:31-19:00	17:31-19:30
V. Excellent	(men)	8:37- 9:40	9:45-10:45	10:00-11:00	10:30-11:30	11:00-12:30	11:15-13:59
	(women)	11:50-12:29	12:30-13:30	13:00-14:30	13:45-15:55	14:30-16:30	16:30-17:30
VI. Superior	(men)	> 8:37	> 9:45	>10:00	>10:30	>11:00	>11:15
	(women)	>11:50	>12:30	>13:00	>13:45	>14:30	>16:30

*< Means "less than"; > means "more than."

AEROBIC TRAINING METHODS

Long, slow distance training (duration)

The oldest and most traditional method of all is simply running, or jogging, long distances at a "slow" rate of speed. The terms "jogging" and "running" are not to be used interchangeably. Jogging may be defined as moving somewhat faster than walking, whereas running implies the maintaining of a specific pace, which forces your heart to work at a greater intensity.

Jogging or running long distances will achieve a higher level of aerobic fitness, provided the duration, intensity and frequency factors are observed. It most certainly is possible to attain an appropriate heart rate, and thus the required intensity, by jogging. The amount of aerobic involvement is the key factor. Without question, the individual who jogs does meet one of the three major training principles, namely the duration principle.

Interval training (intensity)

Rather than jogging or running slowly over long distances, the individual combines various sprints over shorter distances in a specified time period, possibly with a prescribed rest period between each run. This system of training is based on the Swedish training method called "fartlek," actually meaning "speed play." There is an infinite variety of interval training methods. One example used at the Naval Academy will illustrate the interval training method.

It is a physical education requirement for all male midshipmen to run the mile not slower than 6 minutes and 30 seconds. A number of midshipmen train hard and consistently to achieve that goal. One of their training programs is interval training. It is structured in the following manner.

First, midshipmen must carry out an appropriate warmup routine. After a 10- to 15-minute warmup the men will carry out the following interval training: They will run 6 times 440 yards each at 90 seconds; there will be a timed rest period of not more than two minutes. An appropriate interval training is structured for the women as well, with consideration to the fact that women have a mile run requirement of seven minutes and thirty seconds. This training illustrates interval training. There is an infinite variety of interval training routines which can be applied to swimming, cycling and skiing. Without question, the individual does meet a second of the three training principles, namely, the intensity principle.

Alternating hard and easy training (frequency)

No coach would require a team to perform under maximum stress conditions every single day of the athletes' training. The human body must have time to recover after every day of highly intensive training. If this rule is not observed, there will be no progress. It must be understood that any individual who wishes to achieve a better performance in cardiovascular fitness must be willing to train to his point of fatigue and then push through it, continuing to train even though the apparent limits of oxygen capability have already been reached. This type of training causes stress, because the individual continues to make oxygen demands of his body, although the body is unable to take in adequate oxygen supplies. How is such a state possible? It is, because the body is able to tolerate a certain amount of oxygen debt.

Such training is necessary only for those who wish to achieve a high degree of cardiovascular fitness. Such training is not harmful if the individual is already in a highly trained state and is healthy enough to subject his body to that type of stress. It must be noted that such a training day must be followed by a training day where the individual performs well within oxygen reserves. An easy training day must follow a hard training day. Were this principle not observed then the body could not recover and it would not be possible to train a minimum of three to four days a week. Thus, the third training principle, frequency, would not be observed. Aerobic fitness would not be achieved.

At this point in time our reader is ready to select that type of aerobic training exercise that suits him or her best. Undoubtedly the reader understands a basic fact by now. It makes no difference what the activity is that one chooses. It is a matter of personal preference, as long as the frequency, duration and intensity principles are involved.

SELECTING YOUR AEROBIC TRAINING PROGRAM

It is assumed that you have read all material presented so far. It would be a mistake to select a program without that important information. As you select a training program you should be strongly influenced by your health, personal desires and to a certain extent, your age. As the programs are presented, a brief introduction will be given to discuss various aspects of the suggested activity.

Jogging

In the United States there is a prevalent feeling that one simply must jog or run to be fit. As the reader has learned, this simply is not so. In fact, in many cases jogging or running is not desirable because the activity is an event which places a great amount of weight on the skeletal structure. This, in some cases is not desirable because of prior injuries or conditions. Researchers have shown that those who jog or run more than 15 miles a week are more prone to injury. However, this does not mean that jogging and running cannot be highly enjoyable and invigorating activities.

The program outlined below was used by faculty members of the Naval Academy who had no background in jogging.

What: Jogging is running with a slow, easy pace. The runner's foot swings slightly over the point of impact, and returns. The runner lands gently on the ball of his foot, or slightly flatfooted; now the jogger's foot rocks forward from the rear to the ball of his foot; he gently pushes off.

How: Begin by moving slightly faster than a walk. Jog until breathing heavily then walk until breathing becomes normal again; but do not stop-walk instead.

In the beginning stages it is important to avoid oxygen debt, or being winded. Oxygen debt occurs during strenuous exercise. Oxygen is drawn from the body storage for some of the energy. This debt must be repaid. Usually oxygen debt develops after several minutes of vigorous activity; time will vary depending upon the individual.

Course: One complete circuit around our gymnasium deck = one twelfth of a mile.

Thus, one mile = 12 laps.

One complete lap around Farragut = *One mile. Avoid hard surfaces.*

Records: Initially, work indoors; count total laps completed; record quarter-mile segments below. If you walk to rest between jogging laps, keep track of total laps and divide by two. (For ex. You jog 3, walk one, jog 3, walk one, jog 3, walk one = 12 laps completed divided by two = 6 laps, or two quarter-mile segments.)

For each workout, for each quarter mile you complete, place one mark in the appropriate day.

	FIRST DAY	SECOND DAY	THIRD DAY	FOURTH DAY	TOTAL
DATE					
MARKS					
DATE	5th	6th	7th	8th	
MARKS					
DATE	9th	10th	11th	12th	
MARKS					

Records for Jogging Training

Running the mile for time - training

The outlined program is designed for those midshipmen who need to train seriously to meet their mile run requirement in physical education. At this juncture the alert reader may wonder how the duration principle is met if the stipulated training takes less than 35 minutes. The answer is that other activities, such as exercises, or parts of other programs can supplement the total time trained.

Objective: TO RUN THE MILE IN AT LEAST 6:30 MEN, 7:30 WOMEN

Pace: 1st 440 yds. = 87; 88-89 seconds

2nd 440 yds. = 2:58-2:59; 3:00 - 3:10 (anything slower than 3:08 is an indication of trouble)

3rd 440 yds. = 4:33 - 4:43 (anything slower indicates failure)

Training: Your running sessions should always be one of the below:

a. over distance-2 miles +
b. speed work-short, intermittent sprints
c. pace work-learn to run a 440 in exactly 90"

Select any of the five listed workouts shown below:

WORKOUT

Men: To run the mile in 6:30

#1 — Jog three miles, 6 x 60 yards repeated sprints.

#2 — 3 x 880 yards, each in 3:10; rest 6 minutes between each 880
Sprint 8 x 40 yards.

#3 — Jog two miles, twice around Farragut. Sprint 15 x 60 yards.

#4 — Jog five miles.

#5 — 6 x 440 yards, each in 90″ rest 5 minutes between each.

WORKOUT

Women: To run the mile in 7:30

#1 — Jog three miles, 6 x 60 yards, repeat sprints

#2 — 3 x 880 yards, each in 3:35; rest 6 minutes between each 880.
Sprint 8 x 40 yards.

#3 — Jog two miles, twice around Farragut. Sprint 15 x 60 yards.

#4 — Jog five miles.

#5 — 6 x 440 yards, each in 1:45; rest 5 minutes between each.

The above workouts are sample training sessions. They are designed for midshipmen who are in a low state of physical fitness. The five workouts described above should be repeated two or three times. Fifteen workouts should be completed before changes are made.

After three weeks the same workouts can be continued, but the resting interval should be decreased and the number of sprints should be increased.

Remember, do not work out the day before you are tested. Your body must have an opportunity to recover.

Swimming

One of the healthiest of all activities is swimming, the reason being that there is no weight-bearing effect on the skeletal system. Frequently one hears the adage "no pain, no gain." Unfortunately this is misleading. Nobody should train when the pain is the result of sore ligaments, or of a skeletal nature. However, as was described previously, under certain conditions the pain resulting from lack of oxygen should be ignored, if progress is to be made.

Swimming:	BECOME A MEMBER IN THE 25-MILE CLUB IN ONE MONTH.
How:	Swim any comfortable stroke, use a kick-board, and go as far as you comfortably can; when you become stressed, climb out and rest. (Read the information on "oxygen debt" in the jogging information.)
Course:	One width of the Instruction Pool is 20 yards; thus 5½ round trips = 220 yards.
Records:	Count total number of your round trips completed, without resting. Enter each 220-yard segment below. Fractional parts should not be counted. Or, simply record the number of yards each day.

	FIRST DAY	SECOND DAY	THIRD DAY	FOURTH DAY	TOTAL
DATE					
MARKS					
DATE	5th	6th	7th	8th	
MARKS					
DATE	9th	10th	11th	12th	
MARKS					

Records for Swimming Training

Such record keeping is helpful, particularly in the early stages of training. A swimming program of greater intensity is shown below.

Select any of the five listed workouts shown below:

WORKOUT

#1 — 1 X 200 yards, elementary backstroke   : 6 minutes, rest 2 min.
     2 X 400 yards, any stroke . . . . :10 minutes, rest 3 min.

     1 X 200 yards, any stroke . . . . : 4 minutes

#2 — 4 X 300 yards, any stroke . . . . : 7 min. 30 sec., rest 2 min.

#3 — 1 X 1200 yards, any stroke . . . . : 6 minutes

#4 — 1 X 200 yards, elementary backstroke . : 6 minutes, rest 2 min.
     1 X 300 yards, any stroke . . . . : 6 minutes, rest 60 sec.
     1 X 400 yards, any stroke . . . . :10 minutes, rest 2 min.
     1 X 300 yards, any stroke . . . . : 6 minutes, rest 60 sec.
     1 X 200 yards, any stroke . . . . : 3 min. 30 sec., to 4 min.

#5 — 1 X one mile, any stroke . . . . :45 minutes

---

In swimming, just as in any of the other aerobic training programs, it is important to constantly be aware of the three training principles discussed: intensity, frequency and duration.

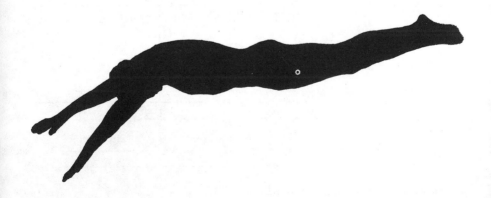

Cycling

Cycling has many advantages. It can be carried out out of doors; the weight-bearing effect is minimal, and there is an endless variety of training courses one might choose.

Frequently one sees cyclists leisurely pedaling along the road. While such an activity is pleasant, there can be no training effect if the intensity principle is not observed. To train appropriately it is necessary to change clothes and wear attire similar to that worn in jogging or running.

Program #1

Cycling:	BECOME A MEMBER IN THE 400-MILE CLUB IN ONE MONTH.
How:	This particular training program is designed for a bicycle with three gears. If you plan to train on a ten-speed, increase the mileage suggested; if you train on a bike without gears, subtract your training dosage. All training principles obviously apply to cycling.
Course:	Select a course which has moderate hills, relatively little traffic and one which is enjoyable to you. You might measure off courses of varying distances. Select three-mile and five-mile courses and possibly a long distance course ranging from ten to twenty miles. You should know the distance you are riding and the time it takes you to cover the stipulated distance.
Records:	Count the total miles covered each training day; record the amount of time required.

Cycling and strength exercises

The suggested push-ups and sit-ups are designed to increase strength. However, when they are combined with an aerobic activity, and are done with the heart rate at the appropriate intensity, they will not only build strength, but continue to increase cardiovascular fitness because the heart rate will not drop below the required training rate. This type of training is demanding. It is obvious that a significant level of cardiovascular fitness must have been reached before such training is attempted. It is suggested that the fit individual train by following the cycling program without exercises one day, and include the strength exercises another.

CYCLING AND STRENGTH EXERCISES

Program #2

Select any of the shown workouts:

WORKOUT

#1 —
a. Warmup: as previously shown
b. Distance: 1 x 12 miles
c. Pace: 4 min. 30 sec. to 5 minute mile pace
d. Exercises: do 30, 40, 50 or 5 less
than maximum push-ups
do 50, 60, 70, or 15 less than
maximum sit-ups
e. Flexibility: train for five minutes to
ten minutes, as shown

#2 —
a. Warmup: as previously shown
b. Distance: 1 x 18, 20, 25 or 30 miles
c. Pace: five minutes each mile, or faster
d. Flexibility: train for five minutes
to ten minutes

#3 —
a. Warmup: as previously shown
b. Distance: 4 x 3 miles
c. Pace: 4 min. 30 sec. to 5-mile pace
d. Exercises: between each set of
cycling three miles,
do 10, 15, 25 or 30 push-ups
do 30, 40, 50 or 60 sit-ups

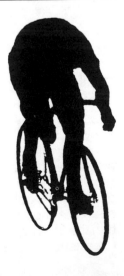

Typical program used by midshipmen at the Naval Academy for cardiovascular conditioning

These routines are of value to midshipmen because they can be carried out under any conditions, without facilities, It is always suggested that some type of softer surface than a steel deck be found when doing sit-ups. The purpose of these exercise routines is to prepare midshipmen to continue to maintain their cardiovascular fitness when going to sea.

CARDIOVASCULAR COMBINED WITH STRENGTH TRAINING
Program #1

The following program is designed to build a sound foundation for cardiovascular fitness. After training four weeks changes can be made to increase requirements. The duration of program #1 must be at least forty minutes.

Jog one-half mile
1 set of jumping jacks (2 minutes-non stop)
Alternate toe touch (1 minute)
Trunk rotation (30 seconds each direction)
440 yards in 90 seconds
30 push-ups
50 sit-ups
440 yards in 90 seconds
40 sitting tucks
30 push-ups
40 sit-ups
30 four-count toe touchers
20 six-count burpees
Wind sprints (2 minutes)
Jog two miles between
14:00 and 15:00 minutes

The alert reader might realize that this type of program could be carried out when away from home on business or vacation.

It is unfortunately a fact that as one ages chronologically there can be no vacation from cardiovascular training. Men and women over thirty-five will begin to realize that regression begins after a layoff of three days.

CARDIOVASCULAR COMBINED WITH STRENGTH TRAINING
Program #2

The following program is the endurance routine familiar to all midshipmen from their Fourth Class Summer PEP program. Modifications have been made so that training can be carried out under shipboard conditions. The photographs shown clarify the described exercises. The duration of Program #2 must be at least forty minutes.

EXERCISES	TIME PERIOD	TRAINING EFFECT
Side straddle hop	90 seconds	warmup and flexibility
Bend and twist	90 seconds	warmup and flexibility
Double arm circles	90 seconds	warmup and flexibility
*Chair-stepping	30 or 60 seconds	leg strength, Increase heart rate
Crawl stroke, forward	90 seconds	flexibility, Increase heart rate
Crawl stroke, backward	90 seconds	flexibility and recovery
Push-ups	20, 25 or 30	pectoral muscles
Sit-ups	20, 30 or 40	abdominal muscles, upper area
Chair-stepping	30 or 60 seconds	leg strength, Increase heart rate
or 220 yard run	40 to 45 seconds	leg strength, Increase heart rate
Alternate left kicks	60 seconds	abdominal muscles, lower area
Flutter kick, front and back	45 seconds, each	lower back and abdominal muscles
*Chair-stepping	30 or 60 seconds	leg strength, Increase heart rate
Explosive jumps	30 or 40 jumps	explosive leg power, Increase heart rate
Side leg raises, right and left	60 seconds, each	leg abductors and recovery
Push-ups	20, 25 or 30	pectoral muscles
Sit-ups	20, 30 or 40	abdominal muscles, upper area
Chair-stepping	30 or 60 seconds	leg strength, Increase heart rate
or 220 yard run	40 or 45 seconds	leg strength, Increase heart rate
Up, out, back and down	45 seconds	lower back muscles and flexibility
Mountain climber	30 seconds	leg and gluteal muscles, heart rate
*Chair-stepping	30 or 60 seconds	leg strength and Increase heart rate
Front leg raises	45 seconds	gluteal muscles and flexibility
Straddle, scissors, hopping	30 seconds, each	leg muscles and recovery
Push-ups	20, 25 or 30	pectoral muscles
Sit-ups	20, 30 or 40	abdominal muscles, upper area
Chair-stepping	30 or 60 seconds	leg strength, Increase heart rate
or 220 yards	40 to 45 seconds	leg strength, Increase heart rate
Sitting-tucks	60 seconds	abdominal muscles, lower area
Bicycle	60 seconds	recovery and flexibility
*Chair-stepping	30 or 60 seconds	leg strength, Increase heart rate
Push-ups	45 seconds, max.	pectoral muscles
*Chair-stepping	30 or 60 seconds	leg strength and Increase heart rate
Sit-ups	1:30, 2:00 or 2:30	abdominal strength, upper area
Chair-stepping	30 or 60 seconds	leg strength and Increase heart rate
or 220 yard run	maximum speed	leg strength and highworking heart rate

*NOTE: include these bench-steps only if a training session of high intensity is desired.

Obviously this program is a highly demanding routine. This routine does not include running. Thus it is possible to carry it out in the smallest of spaces.

CARDIOVASCULAR
CONDITIONING ROUTINES
PROGRAM #2

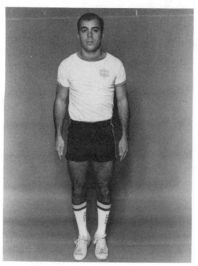 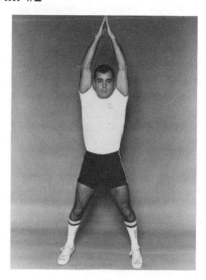

The Side-straddle Hop

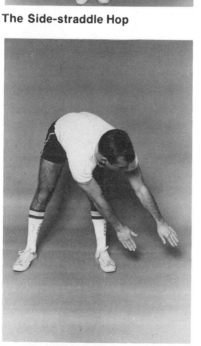 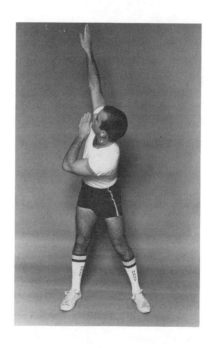

Bending and Twisting

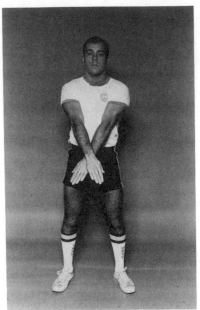 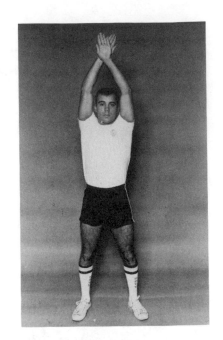

Double Arm Circles

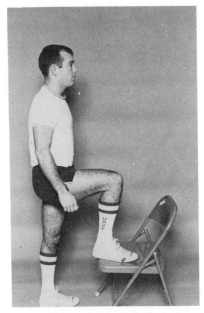 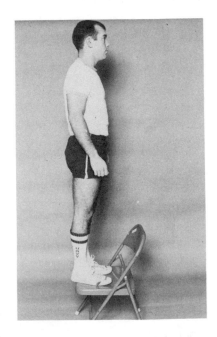

Chair Stepping

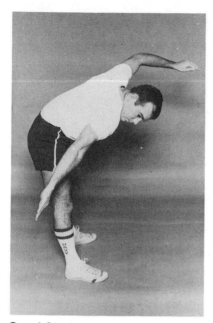

Crawl Stroke, Forward

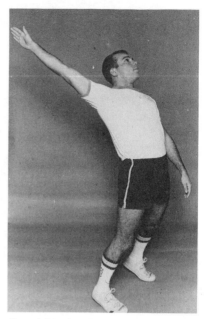

Crawl Stroke, Backward

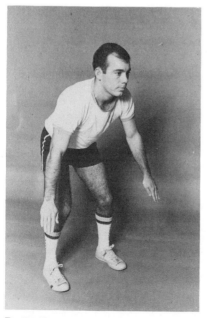

Butterfly

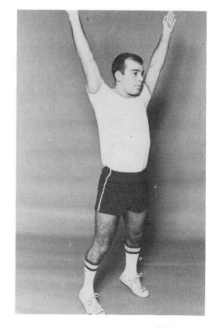

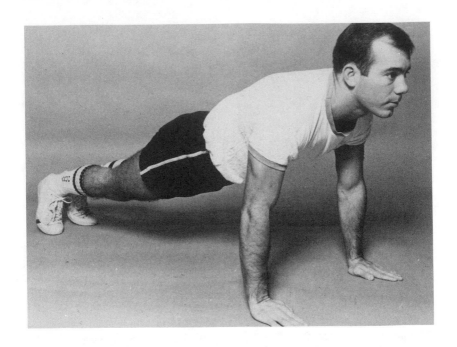

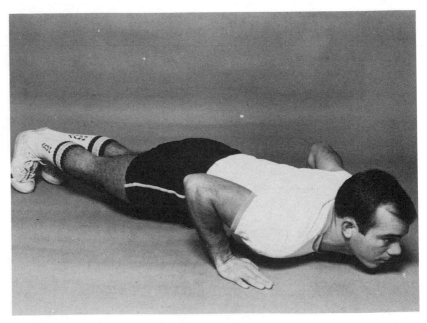

Push-ups

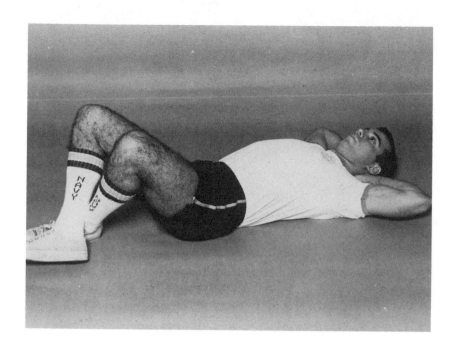

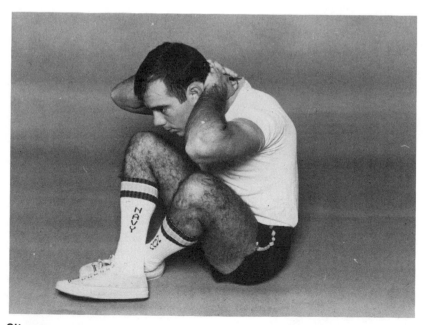

Sit-ups

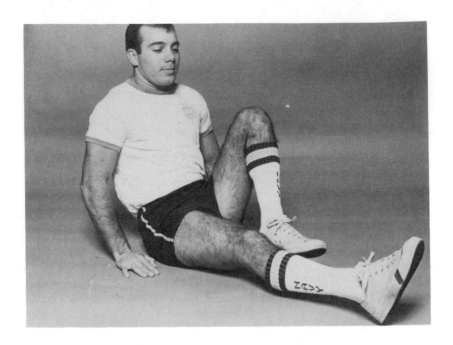

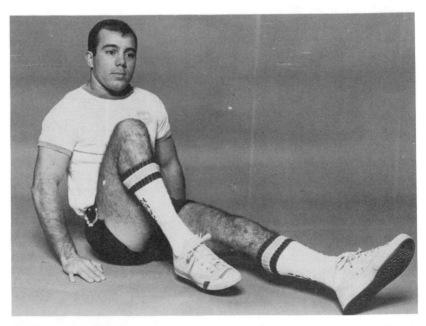

Alternate Leg Kicks

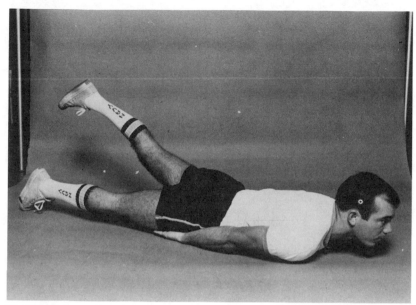

Flutter Kick on Front

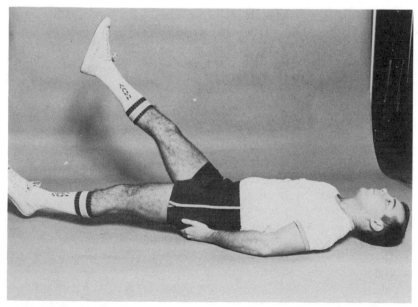

Flutter Kick on Back

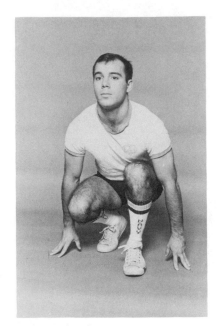 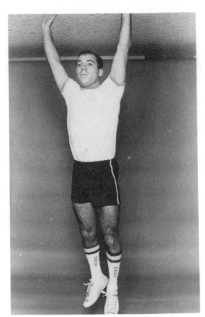

Explosive Jumps

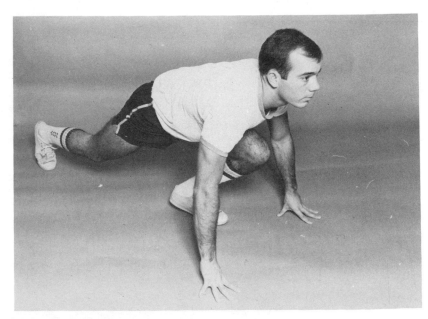

Mountain Climber (alternate legs)

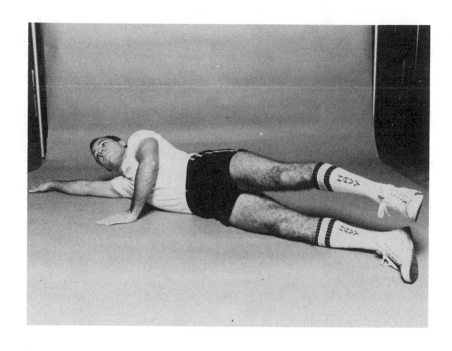

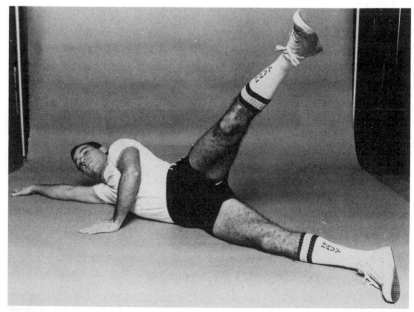

Side Leg Raises

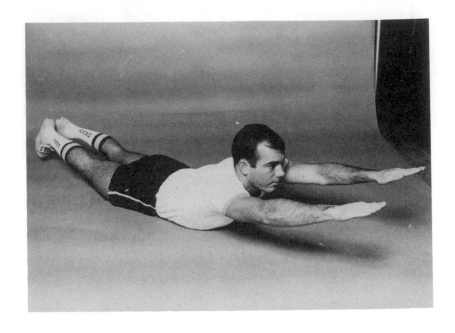

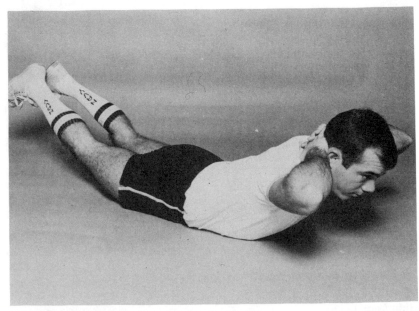

Lower Back Flexibility (up, out, back, down)

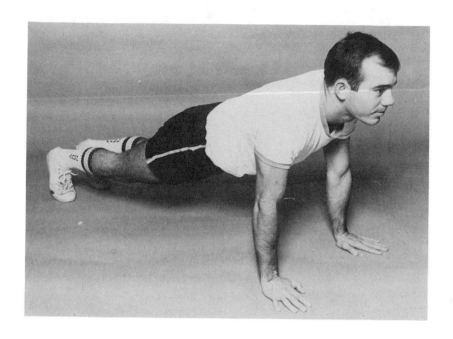

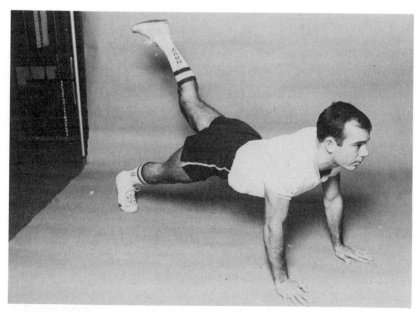

Front Leg Raises

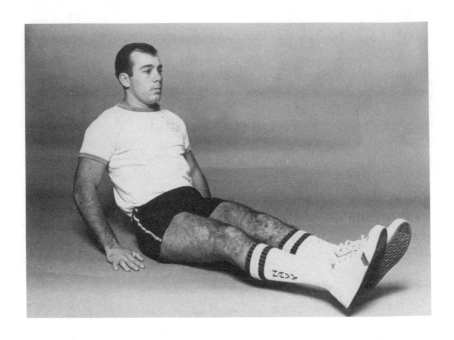

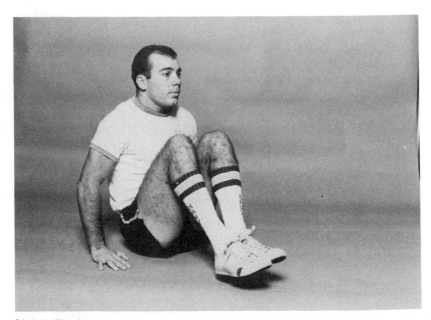

Sitting Tucks

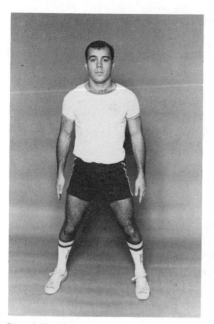

Straddle Hopping

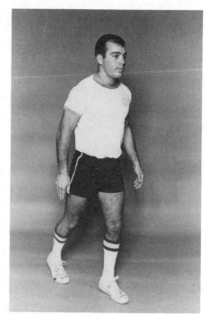

Scissor Hopping

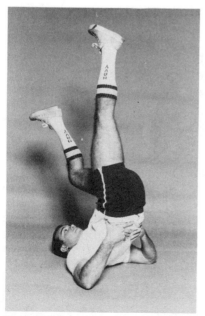

Bicycle

RESULTS OF AEROBIC TRAINING

When individuals are asked why they continue to train aerobically, it has most frequently been the authors' experience to hear the reply, "I feel great after I exercise." Men and women feel better for both physical and psychological reasons, and it is interesting to examine both.

The physical benefits

After individuals have trained for at least six weeks, it becomes obvious that the resting heart rate is reduced. It is known that the heart muscle becomes stronger and becomes more efficient. With each stroke it is able to distribute more blood into the circulatory system; thus a larger number of liters of oxygen is made available for everyday living. Since the number of heartbeats per minute is reduced, the heart gets greater rest between each beat. Energy is conserved. The heart works less during everyday activities. Researchers have determined that there is a decrease in blood pressure, particularly for those who have not already acquired serious cardiovascular problems. In our chapter on nutrition, various aspects of cholesterol are discussed. There is evidence that the type of cholesterol that contributes to heart disease is decreased, whereas the type that protects is increased. But good nutritional habits must accompany sound exercise habits. There can be no question about it—exercise helps control weight. Calories are burned up through aerobic activities. Again, sound nutritional habits must accompany sound aerobic training methods.

Those who exercise aerobically frequently speak of a feeling of well-being which can last from 30 minutes to a period of up to an hour. There are physical reasons for this feeling. During cardiovascular activities carried out at the appropriate level of intensity, secretion of hormones takes place. These hormones, known as endorphins, are released by the pituitary gland. It has been determined by researchers that these endorphins may bring about this feeling of well-being, which can be described as a state of euphoria.

The psychological benefits

In the 1964 Olympic Games, Don Schollander won four gold

medals, a rare feat indeed. After the Olympic Games, Schollander made an interesting statement, which illustrates how mental stress is reduced through physical activity:

> Whether you play a game like squash or tennis, or if you just jog, it's really a form of meditation because you've gotten your mind off your business, or family problems, the world political situation, or anything that may be bothering you. It's a great soul lift. You can escape into your body for a while, and it's like a vacation for your mind.

In 1972 an interesting study was done at the Naval Academy, one designed to investigate the effect of physical activity on brain waves.

It had been established that brain waves displaying high frequency are anxiety-related. In the study midshipmen were asked to carry out physical activity of cardiovascular nature. Brain waves of the men tested were evaluated before and after the exercise. In a significant number of midshipmen, it was noted that high-frequency activity in the brain decreased after exercise. The researcher concludes that since this high-frequency activity appears to be anxiety-related, and exercise can reduce anxiety in individuals."

AFTERWORD

At the Naval Academy we explain to midshipmen that all individuals have a potential maximum level of physical fitness. Because of heredity, interest and training, everyone's maximum level—the 100% level—differs. We point out, however, that it is highly desirable to achieve as high a percentage of the maximum level as possible, and we illustrate our point with the following story:

The Acquired Level of Physical Fitness

0%		40%	50%		80%	100%

Officer A = 40% level	Officer B = 80% level
acquired	acquired

30%	The amount of energy expanded in the work day of both officers

Energy Level Remaining at End of Day: Officer A: 10%
Officer B: 50%

Officer A is not as fit as Officer B. Officer A settled for 40% of his maximum capacity of physical fitness. However, Officer B worked hard and achieved an 80% level of his capacity.

In this model it is assumed that both officers have approximately the same responsibility in their work day and both expand an energy level of 30%. Obviously, at the end of the day Officer A has remaining only a 10% level of his energy; Officer B, however, has 50% of his energy remaining.

Officer A:
1. Arrives home completely exhausted
2. Children want to play with dad—Officer A is too exhausted
3. Wife would like to go out to dinner—Officer A has a drink and is sound asleep ten minutes later

Officer B:
1. Arrives home with a high level of energy
2. Wears out children playing ball
3. Meets wife's needs in any desired manner

We state that Officer B obviously has a much greater zest for living. In addition, it is the hope of the Naval Academy that all graduates will be like Officer B, and not like Officer A.

REFERENCES

1. Pollock, M. J. "Run, Walk, Jog — What's the Difference?", *Medical World News*; May 19, 1972, p. 75.
2. de Vries, H. A. *Physiology of Exercise for Physical Education and Athletics*; Wm. C. Brown Company, Dubuque, Iowa, 1966, p. 78.
3. Katch, F. L., and McArdle, W. D. *Nutrition, Weight Control, and Exercise*; Houghton Mifflin Company, Boston, 1977.
4. Department of the Navy. "OPNAVINST 6110. 1A"; Office of the Chief of Naval Operations, Washington, DC 20350, 17 July 1980.
5. Cooper, K. H. *The Aerobics Program for Total Well Being*; M. Evans and Company, Inc., New York, 1982.

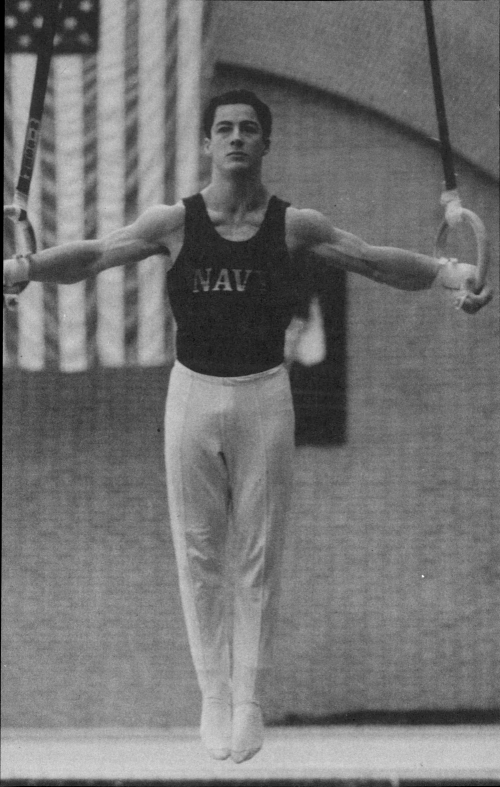

3

MUSCULAR FITNESS —STRENGTH AND ENDURANCE

The truest success is but the development of self.

—Charles Atlas

OBJECTIVES

- Describe the history of strength training.
- Define the terms "muscular strength" and "muscular endurance".
- Cite why training for muscular fitness is important.
- Discuss how muscles function; show where major muscle groups are located and show their function.
- Discuss principles to be considered when training for muscular fitness.
- Give examples of weight training with free weights and commercial weight training machines.
- List for each type of weight equipment procedures to establish starting weights and record keeping.
- Cite benefits of muscular fitness training.

WEIGHT TRAINING THROUGH THE AGES

It certainly is not difficult to trace the development of weight training. Wrestlers and well-developed athletes are seen in sculptures and paintings by Egyptian and Greek artists. One well-known early weight lifter was Milo of Crotona, first to demonstrate the fact that weight training must be carried out on a progressive basis. This athlete lifted a calf several times a week. As the calf grew, Milo's muscles adapted to the increased weight requirement, and as legend presents it, he became the only man capable of lifting a fully-developed ox—a result of his continued progressive weight training.

This legend illustrates a most important principle of strength training—training must be carried out regularly, and the muscles must be exposed to increasingly heavier weights.

People have constantly sought devices to assist them in their training. Objects resembling dumbbells were used by Greeks and in the 1600s by the British. It is said that early weight trainers in England removed clappers from bells and mounted them on hammer handles or pieces of wood. It is believed that this is how the term "dumbbell" originated. Strong men have always appeared in circuses and fairs. In all probability weight lifting became better known as the result of the first modern Olympic Games in Athens in 1896. The Olympic movement has contributed to increased interest in weight lifting.

Unfortunately those who trained with weights carried out their training in basements, unventilated spaces, frequently in areas with inadequate lighting. Few sound training principles were known, and those which were known were not followed. Professional strong men and competitive weight lifters were frequently, and rightfully, accused of being "muscle bound." Little wonder that weight training rapidly fell into disrepute, and that coaches suggested to athletes that weight training not be included in their training.

In the late 1940s T. L. DeLorme, a U.S. Army physician working with soldiers requiring physical rehabilitation, introduced new techniques and documented training principles with weights. As a result training with weights began to be increasingly more accepted, first by physicians, and later by physical educators and coaches.

Today the many values of weight training are soundly supported by research and obvious results.

Why train for muscular fitness?

Survival For military men and women, an adequate level of muscular strength and endurance is vital. Regardless of an aviator's level of cardiovascular fitness and swimming ability, if his plane goes down, he may first of all require muscular strength to pull himself out of a burning cockpit. At sea, aboard ship, there are many instances when an adequate level of muscular strength and endurance is needed simply to carry out the tasks at hand.

Sports performance improvement Every successful coach is fully aware of the significant contribution a proper weight training program makes to the success of his team. Track and field performances have improved in part because of weight training. Some swimming coaches are also using heavy weight training in conjunction with their water training to lower their swimmer's times. College football coaches have recently augmented their staffs by employing strength coaches who have the sole responsibility of increasing muscular strength and endurance for the team.

Appearance Midshipmen frequently undertake a muscular strength training program, not because they are deficient in their strength tests, but simply because they are dissatisfied with their appearance and seek improvement. One young man recently stated it clearly: "When I stand in front of a mirror without clothes on, I don't even like my own body. How can a girl possibly like it?" He was motivated. Psychologists have for a long time explained to us that our self-image is highly important in how we face the world. We designed a muscular strength and endurance program that would without question improve this midshipman's total appearance.

Muscular fitness defined

This aspect of physical fitness is composed of two elements, muscular strength and muscular endurance.

Muscular strength is defined as the ability of the skeletal muscles to exert maximum force against a given external resistance.

Muscular endurance is the body's ability to sustain repeated muscular effort, without diminished efficiency, for as long a time period as possible.

MUSCLES—HOW THEY WORK

Muscle composition

Muscles are composed of thousands of fibers. Weight training may not increase the number of muscle fibers, but it does increase each fiber's diameter. These increases in the size of the fibers bring about a gain in work capability, because the larger muscles can accomplish more. A muscle may simply be considered a family of fibers which have the ability to contract. The fibers are held together by a sheath of connective tissue, muscles are attached to bones by tendons, and the bones are connected by ligaments.

There are 434 voluntary muscles in the body, and these are responsible for all movements a human being can carry out. The action of the muscles attached to the bones provides a mechanical system of levers, the efficiency of which is primarily determined by the strength of the muscles.

Research has demonstrated that muscle growth takes place primarily when the muscle is exercised anaerobically. This means that if maximum strength development is to take place in each exercise, the muscles must be fatigued by executing the stipulated number of repetitions within sixty seconds. To achieve maximum muscle growth, the weight training must involve as great a mass of muscle fibers as possible.

Research has shown that at least eight repetitions must be executed before the majority of the muscle fibers are fatigued. During the contractions, chemical reactions take place in the muscle providing the fuel for the muscles to contract. When all fibers are recruited, muscular failure (fatigue) takes place. Unless such failure takes place within sixty seconds, the muscle will require oxygen to continue its work. Thus, the exercise becomes aerobic (training with oxygen) instead of anaerobic (training without oxygen).

MUSCLES—SEX FACTORS

It has been well documented by researchers that women's response to weight training is similar to that of men.[2][3][5][7][8] Essentially these researchers have demonstrated that the percentage of increase in strength for women in all muscle groups except one—arm muscles—was the same or better than in men. It must be remembered, however, that some gains made by women are probably because women had lower initial levels of strength than men by virtue of cultural differences, as pointed out by Cox and Lenz.[5] However, the fear that weight training will develop bulky, mannish, overly-muscled women is unfounded. In fact, the opposite—a trim, firm well-contoured figure—is usually found among women who train regularly in strength-developing routines. An excellent example is the appearance of world-class women gymnasts, who probably are among the strongest of all women.

Westcott has demonstrated[7] that weight training increases the muscle size of men to far greater a degree than in women, and it has been shown that this is due to the male sex hormone, testosterone, which determines the size of the muscles. As a result of genetic composition men have a greater capability to develop muscle size and strength than women. However, it is beginning to be discovered that women can develop excellent levels of strength, provided adequate training takes place. This is shown in the improvement of women midshipmen in pull-ups (Table 3.1).

Performance in Pull-ups by Women Midshipmen 1979-1983

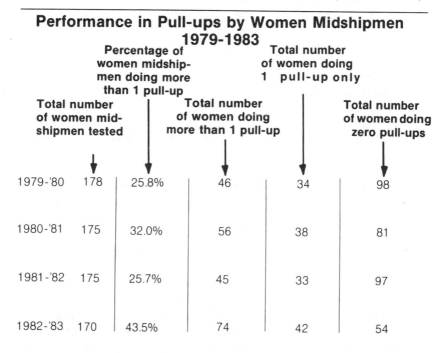

Total number of women midshipmen tested	Percentage of women midshipmen doing more than 1 pull-up	Total number of women doing more than 1 pull-up	Total number of women doing 1 pull-up only	Total number of women doing zero pull-ups
1979-'80 178	25.8%	46	34	98
1980-'81 175	32.0%	56	38	81
1981-'82 175	25.7%	45	33	97
1982-'83 170	43.5%	74	42	54

Table 3.1

Table 3.1 appears to indicate that the number of women unable to do pull-ups is decreasing. Also, it is noted that the percentage of women midshipmen able to do more than one pull-up has increased from 25.8% in 1980 to 43.5% in 1983.

There is no question about it: In both sexes, muscles respond to training. They adapt to the demands made upon them by the owner. Unless appropriate training principles are observed, however, results may well be unsatisfactory.

TRAINING FOR MUSCULAR FITNESS

Misconceptions

In our physical fitness classes, when we ask midshipmen to list the important principles to be considered when training for muscular strength and endurance, the following are most frequently listed:

- lifting heavy weights for a muscular appearance
- spending long periods of time training
- special nutrition and additional protein intake
- training with the right type of equipment

It becomes obvious that each of these points is a misconception and must be rectified.

Training principles

Muscular appearance If a midshipman has such a goal as his primary objective, it is important to understand that it is not a question of following a certain program, but rather of heredity. One is not able to compete successfully for the "Mr. America" title if one does not happen to have inherited the right genes from one's parents.

It is entirely conceivable that two midshipmen will follow precisely the same training program. Yet one will begin to look like Atlas, whereas his training partner will gain strength and improve his appearance, but will not look at all like his more fortunate partner, who happened to have the right parents.

Quality, not quantity Coaches and athletes seek maximum performances. This is logical. Such an approach to weight training is counter-productive, however. Weight trainers must concentrate on correct execution and technique rather than the amount of weight lifted in any exercise. If there is too heavy a weight load, it becomes necessary for other muscle groups to assist, with the result that the muscles being trained will not get appropriate emphasis because of muscle substitution. Thus the necessary point of fatigue is not attained by the primary muscle group in training.

The key to gaining strength is not the amount of weight that is lifted, but the correct execution of the lift. It is possible for two midshipmen to have precisely the same program. One midshipman might be precise and carry out all exercises with correct technique. The other might not. Research has shown that the individual training incorrectly experiences significantly less success than the individual who is training correctly.

Length of training time Weight trainers who spend endless periods of time are not training efficiently. The key is to select a series of appropriate exercises and then to carry out the training with correct execution. Such a training program need not take longer than 30 minutes, depending on the program design.

Nutrition and no additional protein Readers will find extensive information on this subject in the nutrition chapter in Part II. At this time, however, it is useful to state that no special nutritional practices contribute to better performances or gains in weight training. Research has shown that regardless of size and physical activity, the body has a fixed protein requirement, which may be simply stated as follows: For every kilogram (2.2 pounds) of body weight, one gram of protein is needed every twenty-four-hour period. There is little question about it. Most Americans do not need to take additional protein just because they are training hard with weights. The only individuals who grow stronger because of additional protein intake are the manufacturers, who have to carry their heavy money bags to the bank.

The "right" type of equipment Every reader must understand that the type of equipment has little to do with results unless the equipment is used correctly. Strength gains can be achieved by training with Nautilus machines, Universal machines, barballs, or any of the commercial equipment available. The key is correct execution of the exercises. There will be little gain if correct technique is not enforced and if specific training principles are not observed.

ADDITIONAL KEY TRAINING PRINCIPLES

Momentary muscular failure

Physiologically speaking, the human organism adapts to stress, and our muscular system is no exception. Muscular growth takes place when additional work is required of the muscle, even though its energy limits have been reached. If work demands continue, muscular failure will take place, and it is important that such failure be achieved within sixty seconds or less, for then optimum conditions for growth and strength development are created. If the muscle is allowed to rest momentarily, and is then again forced to work, energy demands will be met aerobically and not chemically. Aerobic training will contribute to cardiovascular fitness, but in weight training the goal is muscular strength and muscular endurance; thus, the purpose is defeated if momentary failure is not induced within sixty seconds.

Speed of execution

A great deal has been written about the speed with which an exercise should be done. The supporters of the Universal Gym machine have always stressed that exercises should be done explosively. It is argued that many athletic events require explosiveness. Examples are the shot put, the charge of a lineman in football, and the kicking of a soccer ball. On the other hand, supporters of Nautilus equipment have explained that explosiveness creates a ballistic effect, which is not conducive to strength building. (But we should note that it is almost impossible to carry out exercises on the Nautilus machines explosively.) The reader should understand that all exercises consist of two phases. First there is the positive phase, in which the weight is lifted. Then comes the second phase—the negative aspect—when the weight is lowered. Obviously gravity makes the lowering easier.

The speed with which to do the positive lift has been discussed above. According to the Universal theory, each execution should be done explosively. "Think speed" is the key slogan. The Nautilus theory says that the weight should be lifted positively to a count of two. The negative phase, when gravity helps, is a most important aspect of training and should be done very slowly, preferably to a count of four. It is necessary to counteract gravity. This negative phase has proven to build strength to an even greater degree than the positive aspect.

Lifting through the full range of motion This most important principle had been ignored in early weight training days. Weight lifters were considered to be "muscle-bound," unable to perform functions of flexibility simply because that aspect of their training was ignored. Lifters consistently failed to train the muscle through the full range of motion. Little wonder that the muscles grew less flexible and weight training was considered a failure.

Flexibility can be simply illustrated by lifting both arms later-ally over the head until the palms touch. If the palms are not touching, the activity is not carried out through the full range of motion. When a lifter finds it impossible to lift through the full range of motion, the amount being trained with should be reduced. If that does not bring about full range of motion, then it is probably due to an existing lack of flexibility. By being conscious of lifting through as much of the range of motion as possible, flexibility will begin to be restored, maintained and improved.

Frequency of training

It has been demonstrated that the most gain will be made if an individual trains every other day. Most studies indicate that opti-mum muscular growth takes place if a rest period of 48 hours is permitted. While there would be no harm in training daily, it should be clear that for the time invested, maximum growth takes place if a 48-hour rest period is part of the training system. It might be desirable to plan to train every other day. The serious weight trainer should not permit more than a two-day rest from time to time. If there is more than a two-day rest, strength loss occurs.

Training with a partner

It is desirable to find a partner when training with weights. The lift-er must achieve momentary failure in the muscle group being trained, but it is most difficult to exert effort to that great an extent unless a partner is present to urge the lifter on to achieve an all-out effort.

A partner is also helpful in checking technique. A partner will suggest reducing or increasing the training load depending on the lifter's performance. In addition, a partner can easily change the amount of weight being lifted on machines such as the Nauti-lus and Universal.

Another important reason for having a partner is to ensure safety, particularly if the individual trains with free weights. In such a case a training partner is indispensable.

Training sequence

The order in which muscles are exercised is important. The larger muscles of the body should be trained first, then the smaller groups. If the smaller muscle is exhausted first, it cannot act as a stabilizer of the larger muscle group as that one is exposed to maximum load. This principle is taken into consideration when weight training rooms, such as Nautilus rooms, are arranged.

MAJOR MUSCLE GROUPS— LOCATION AND FUNCTION

The locations, names, and functions of the major muscle groups are listed on the following pages.

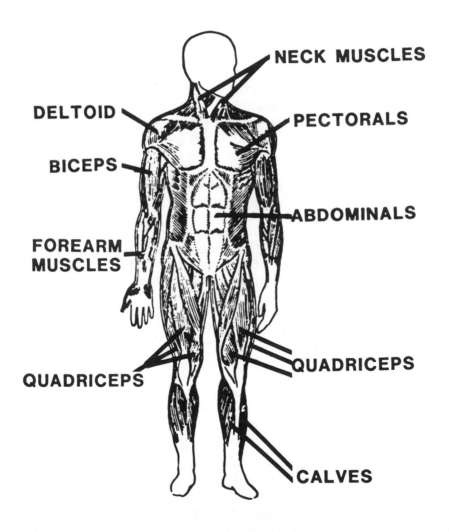

NECK MUSCLES

DELTOID

PECTORALS

BICEPS

ABDOMINALS

FOREARM MUSCLES

QUADRICEPS

QUADRICEPS

CALVES

Front view

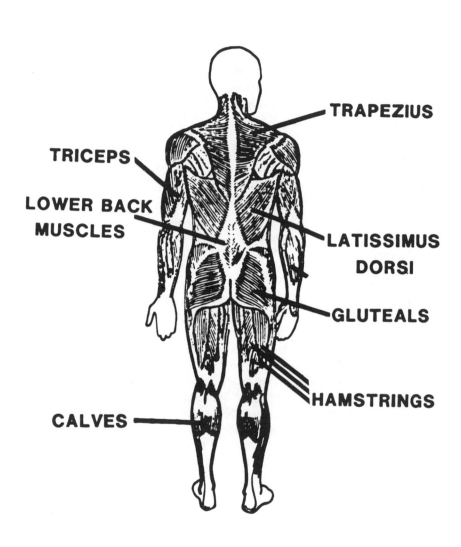

Rear view

Also, the training sheet from the Universal system works the bigger muscles before the smaller ones.

Warmup The purpose of warming up the body is to prepare it for intensive exercise. It is important to saturate the muscles with blood, increase the body temperature, increase the working heart rate and alert the nervous system. These preliminaries increase performance and reduce the risk of injury.

To accomplish an adequate warmup the reader is directed to the preceding chapter, on cardiovascular fitness; there on page 43 are described warmup exercises. Next the weight trainer is encouraged to carry out one set of his weight-training routine, with only one-half the amount of weight that will be used when the actual training for strength begins.

Breathing It is important to breathe continuously while training with weights. It is a serious mistake to hold one's breath while straining to complete a repetition, for in this case the training individual closes off the blood flow to an area of the body. Such action may well increase pressure in the chest and interfere with venous blood return to the heart, and a significant rise in blood pressure is the result. This entire undesirable condition, resulting from breath-holding, is known as the Valsalva Response.

Midshipmen frequently ask when to breathe in and out. It is most desirable to exhale when maximum stress is assigned to the muscles. We tell midshipmen to follow a simple rule: "Always blow the weight up." This rule is applicable for any possible weight exercise if the weight is pressed from the shoulders, for example, over the head, the weight goes up. Thus, exhaling occurs while the weight goes up. The key factors are to breathe regularly and continuously. Breathing is a natural process.

Repetitions A single weight training repetition is moving a weight through the full range of motion and includes positive and negative action. Often repetitions are called "reps" by weight trainers.

Sets A strength training routine may consist of eight to twelve different exercises, so that all muscle groups will be trained. When all exercises of the training routine have been completed, one set has been carried out. If strength training is done properly, one set is as beneficial in achieving strength gains as multiple sets.

Buttocks and legs

1) Gluteals: The gluteal muscles are the largest and strongest muscle group of the body. These three muscles—the gluteus minimus, medius, and maximus—form the buttocks.
   a. Function—The gluteal muscles extend the hip in such activities as running and jumping.
   b. Training—Barbell squat, leg press, Nautilus hip and back machine.

2) Quadriceps: The quadriceps group is the largest and strongest muscle group of the leg, located on the front of the thigh. This group is composed of four muscles: the rectus femorsi, vastus medialis, vastus lateralis, and vastus intermedius.
   a. Function—The quadriceps extends the lower leg in activities involving running, jumping and kicking.
   b. Training—Squat, leg extention, leg press.

3) Hamstring: The hamstrings are the antagonistic muscle group of the quadriceps, located on the back of the upper leg. When weight lifting for the legs, many athletes exercise the quadriceps exclusively with little regard for the hamstrings. This leads to a weak hamstring area and often results in injury.
   a. Function—While the quadriceps extends the lower leg, the hamstrings flex it. Running, jumping and kicking all use the hamstrings.
   b. Training—Squat, leg curls, leg press.

4) Calves: Calf muscles are located on the back side of the lower leg.
   a. Function—Calf muscles such as the gastrocnemius serve in the extention of the foot in activities like running, jumping or tumbling.
   b. Training—Calf raise, toe press.

Torso

1) Latissimus dorsi: The latissimus dorsi is located on the upper back and is the largest muscle group of the upper body.
   a. Function—The primary function of the latissimus dorsi is to perform pulling motions such as pull-ups, rope climb, or the crawl stroke in swimming.
   b. Training—Pull-ups, bent-over rowing, pullovers, lat pull down.

2) Lower back muscles:
   a. Function—Lower back muscles straighten the torso to an upright position.
   b. Training—Squat, good mornings, hyperextentions, Nautilus hip and back machine.

3) Deltoids: The deltoid is a triangluar-shaped muscle that covers the shoulder.
   a. Function—Deltoid muscles are responsible for extending the arm forward, sideways or upward in such activities as throwing, reaching or punching.
   b. Training—Military press, lateral raise, upright rowing, Nautilus double shoulder machine.

4) Trapezius: The trapezius muscles are located on the upper back and neck area.
   a. Function—These muscles raise the shoulders upward, and protect the neck from injury in sports such as football and wrestling.
   b. Training—Shoulder shrug, Nautilus neck and shoulder machine.

5) Pectorals: The pectorals are composed of two muscles, the pectoralis major and minor. These muscles combine to form a large flat area that stretches across the front of the chest.
   a. Function—Extending the arms in pressing actions such as performing push-ups.
   b. Training—Bench press, flies, Nautilus double chest machine.

6) Abdominals: Many muscles combine to form the abdominals, located on the stomach. Abdominal muscles often act as stabilizers for many sports activities and weight-training exercises.
   a. Function—Abdominal muscles contract the body from an extended position.
   b. Training—Sit-ups, leg raises.

Arms
1) Triceps: Three muscles combine to form the triceps, making it the largest muscle group of the arm. The triceps is located on the back region of the upper arm.
   a. Function—The triceps extends the forearm in motions like throwing, batting and performing dips.
   b. Training—Triceps extension, French curl, behind the back dips.

2) Biceps: The biceps consists of two muscles and is located on the front of the upper arm.
   a. Function—The biceps is chiefly involved in pulling motion like rope climb or chin-ups. The latissimus dorsi and biceps often assist each other.
   b. Training—Biceps curl, chin-ups.

3) Forearm muscles:
   a. Function—Gripping and flexing the wrist in activities like golf, tennis and baseball are the primary function of forearm muscles.
   b. Training—Wrist curls, wrist rolls.

MUSCULAR TRAINING METHODS

It is possible to train for muscular strength and endurance with various equipment.

EXERCISES BY MUSCLE GROUP AND EQUIPMENT

	Free weights	Multi-station equipment	Nautilus equipment
Gluteal and erector spinae group	squat stiff-legged deadlift	leg press hyperextension	hip and back hip abduction leg press
Quadriceps	squat	leg extension leg press	leg extension leg press
Hamstrings	squat	leg curl leg press	leg curl leg press
Abductor group	squat	leg press	hip abduction
Gastroc, and soleus group	calf raise	toe press on leg press	calf-raise on multi-exercise toe press on leg press
Latissimus dorsi	bent-over rowing bent-arm pullover stiff-arm pullover	chin-up pull down on lat machine	pullover behind neck torso/arm chin-up on multi-exercise
Trapezius	shoulder shrug dumbbell shoulder shrug	shoulder shrug	neck and shoulder rowing torso

EXERCISES BY MUSCLE GROUP AND EQUIPMENT, Cont.

	Free weights	Multi-Station equipment	Nautilus equipment
Pectoralis majors	bench press dumbbell fly	bench press parallel dip	double chest 1. arm cross 2. decline press parallel dip on multi-exercise
Biceps	standing curl	curl chin-up	compound curl biceps curl multi curl
Triceps	triceps extension	press down on	triceps extension
Forearm group	wrist curl	wrist curl	wrist curl on multi-exercise
Abdominal and oblique group	sit-up side bend with dumbbell	sit-up leg raise	abdominal rotary torso side bend on multi-exercise
Neck group	neck bridge (dangerous)	neck harness	4-way neck rotary neck neck and shoulder

From Darden, Ellington: Strength Training Principles: How to Get the Most Out of Your Workouts. Winter Park, Fla: Anna Publishing Co., Fall. 1977.

Training with free weights We suggest the following procedure to midshipmen. Our readers may use the suggestions and record-keeping chart as a model.

1. Become familiar with the training principles discussed in this chapter. Consult the major muscle group charts and tables and select six to eight exercises which will train all muscle groups.

2. Enter the names of the exercises selected on your Personal Record Chart (shown on the next page).

3. Find a partner and establish your starting weight for each of the exercises indicated on the chart. Note, the initial number of repetitions has already been entered (R = repetitions); when you have established your starting weight according to directions on the chart, enter the starting weight in the space marked W.

4. If you are not sure how to do the various exercises, consult the drawings and descriptions on the pages following the Record Chart.

MIDSHIPMEN RECORD CARD

Last Name, First Name, Initial   Cl. Co.   Starting Date   Body weight
Equipment: FREE WEIGHTS

Exercises	Date W/R	Date W/R	Date W/R	Date W/R	Date W/R	Date W/R
1. DEAD LIFT	12					
2. HALF-SQUAT	12					
3. TOE RAISES	12					
4. BARBELL PRESS	8					
5. BENCH PRESS	8					
6. STANDING CURL	8					
7. BARBELL BENT ROWING	8					
8. SIT-UPS (weight behind head)	12					

TO ESTABLISH STARTING WEIGHTS:

a. For exercises 4, 5, 6 and 7 — whatever you can lift COMFORTABLY AND CORRECTLY, 6 times.

b. For exercises 1, 2, 3 and 8 — whatever you can lift COMFORTABLY AND CORRECTLY, 10 times.

TRAIN PROGRESSIVELY: Observe the range shown below.

RANGE: If you begin with 8 repetitions go from 8–12 repetitions. If you begin with 10 repetitions go from 12–16 repetitions.

When you reach the top of the range, increase your weight load slightly and begin at the beginning of the range.

ADDITIONAL TRAINING POINTS AS REMINDERS

a. BREATHING: Breathe regularly, never hold your breath, blow the weight up.

b. ADVANCED TRAINING: After a foundation has been built lifters may progress to heavier weights and fewer repetitions. IT TAKES SIX WEEKS TO BUILD A MINIMAL FOUNDATION.

c. NUTRITIONAL AIDS AND VITAMINS: These are not necessry for progress.

d. WARMUP: (a) Use the exercises described in Chapter II, or jog one-half mile very slowly.

(b) Work through your training routine at one-half your regular training load on this record card.

FREE WEIGHT EXERCISES

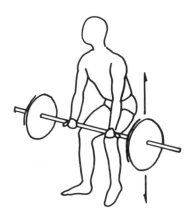

Exercise 1: Dead Lift

Muscles Trained
Quadriceps, hamstrings, lower back muscles.

Description of Exercise
- Squat behind the barbell.
- Hands are shoulder-width apart; one hand forward, one hand backward.
- Lift the bar by straightening knees and hips.
- When the barbell is in motion, the back begins to become erect.
- When erect, pause momentarily, and return barbell to floor rapidly.

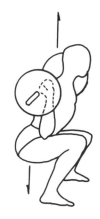

Exercise 2: Half-Squat
Muscles Trained
Quadriceps, hamstrings, calf.

Description of Exercise
- Partner lifts bar and places it across shoulders. (A rack may also be used.)
- Hands are shoulder-width apart.
- Lower body slowly so that thighs are not quite parallel to ground.
- Return to standing position.
- Head up—back straight *always*.

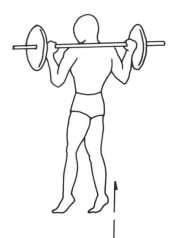

Exercise 3: Rise on Toes
Muscles Trained
Calves.

Description of Exercise
- Lift heels off ground as far as possible. Hold momentarily and lower heels to ground.

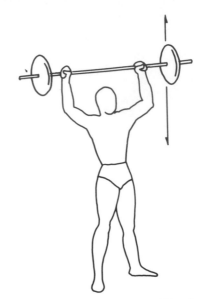

Exercise 4: Press
Muscles Trained
Deltoids, trapezius, triceps.

Description of Exercise
- Bar is brought to shoulders and lies across them. (Begin with dead lift) bar continues to be pulled up until elbows are as high as possible; swing elbows forward; support the bar for starting position.
- Press bar straight up overhead, arms fully extended.
- Momentarily hold bar and slowly return to starting position.
- *Back remains straight. Do not lean. Do not arch.*

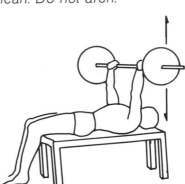

Exercise 5: Bench Press
Muscles Trained
Pectorals, deltoids, triceps.

Description of Exercise
- Lift bar from standard or have partner assist in bringing the bar up at full arms' extension.
- Shoulders, back and gluteus maximus always make contact with bench.
- Slowly lower bar to chest and again extend arms, but do not lock elbows.
- *Do not rest at top of lift.*

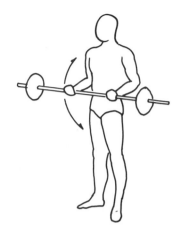

Exercise 6: Curl
Muscles Trained
Biceps.

Description of Exercise
- Hold barbell at full arms' extension; use underhand grip.
- Keep upper arm position unchanged.
- Keep elbow position unchanged.
- Raise barbell until arms are *completely* flexed.
- Slowly lower barbell to initial position.
- *Do not substitute muscles by arching back.*

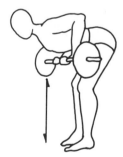

Exercise 7: Rowing
Muscles Trained
Latissimus dorsi, biceps, deltoids.

Description of Exercise
- Keep back parallel to floor.
- Barbell is at full arms' extension.
- Lift bar to chest, pause for a moment and slowly lower bar.
- A wide or narrow grip may be used. (A wider grip puts greater emphasis on the latissimus dorsi.)

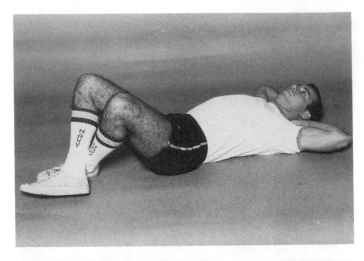

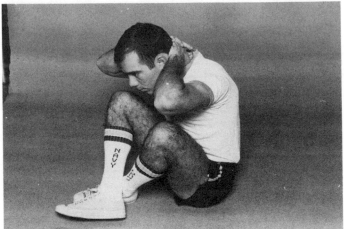

Exercise 8: Sit-Up
Muscles Trained
Abdominals, hip flexors.

Description of Exercise
- Lie back on floor.
- Place a weight in your hand and hold it behind your neck.
- Cross your feet over.
- Sit up until your head breaks the plane of your knees.
- Slowly return to the starting position.
- It is possible to hold the weight on the chest. (Not shown in photograph.)

Training with multi-station equipment We suggest that an individual who has not trained with weights begin with a multi-station machine such as the Universal Gym. It is easier to train on such machines because one need not be concerned with balance, which could cause an inexperienced trainer problems. Also, it is easier to carry out training with proper technique on a machine such as the Universal. We instruct midshipmen to initiate training by using a record sheet similar to the one shown below. The procedure is quite similar.

Name_____ Starting date_____ Body weight_____
Equipment Universal Gym

Exercises	Date W/R	Date W/R	Date W/R	Date W/R	Date W/R	Date W/R	Date W/R	Date W/R
Leg extension								
Leg press								
Leg curl								
Toe press								
Lat pull down								
Bench press								
Shoulder press								
Biceps curl								
Triceps extension								
Wrist curl								
Sit-ups								

THE UNIVERSAL GYM

Many Universal Gyms are equipped with a variable resistance mechanism. This mechanism is effective by changing the fulcrum of the movement arm, allowing the resistance to increase throughout the lift. In most instances one becomes stronger in the mid-range of an exercise, because the body limbs have the mechanical advantage. The variable resistance mechanism is designed to fatigue the muscle through the full range of movement.

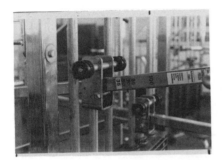 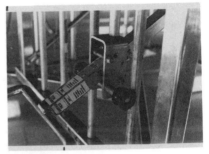

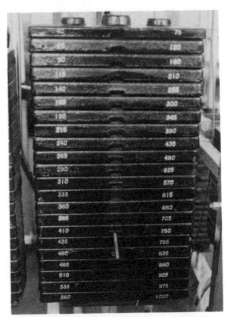

UNIVERSAL'S VARIABLE RESISTANCE

Leg extension

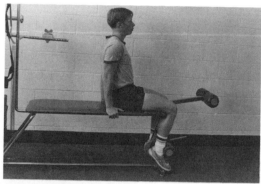

Starting position

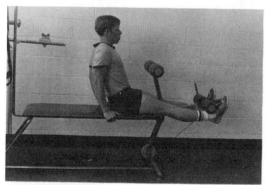

Extended position

Muscles trained: quadriceps

Seated on leg extension machine, the hands grasp the seat slightly behind the buttocks. Extend legs to the straight position, pause momentarily and return to the starting position.

Key Points:

- There is a tendency to perform this exercise too quickly. The positive phase should take 2 seconds and the negative 4 seconds.
- Legs should be extended completely to ensure a full range of motion.

Leg curl

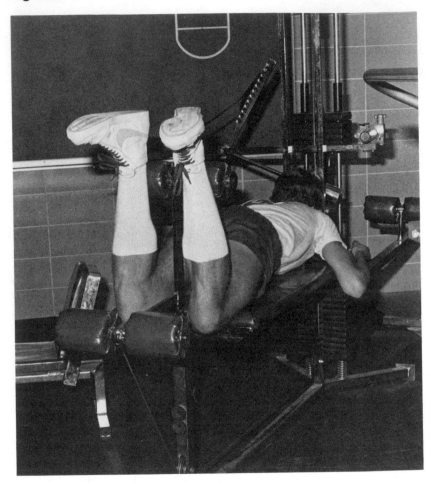

Muscles trained: hamstrings

Lie face down on bench so that your knees are slightly over the edge. Lift heels as high as possible, pause and lower to starting position.

Key Points:

- Legs should be lifted at least perpendicular to floor.
- Do not pull with arms.

Leg press

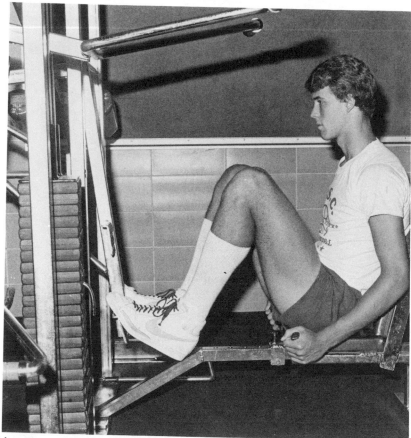

Muscles trained: gluteals, quadriceps, hamstrings

Place feet on the center of foot pedals. Adjust seat so that the knees are bent about 90°. Extend the legs just short of the locked position, pause momentarily and return to the starting position.

Key points:

- Do not allow legs to lock out. This will prevent muscle fiber from resting.
- Keep buttocks in contact with seat at all times.
- Do not let weights bounce prior to each lift. The weight should be *lifted* not bounced.

Toe press

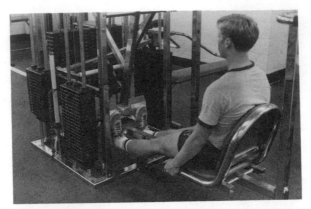

Starting position

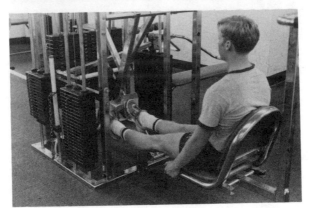

Extended position

Muscles trained: calves

Enter leg press station and place top half of foot on the pedals. Push legs to a locked position. Extend the foot completely, pause and recover to the starting position without bending knees.

Key points:

- Do not bend knees.
- Concentrate on full range.

Lat pull-down

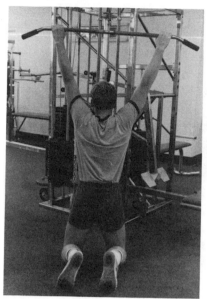

Starting position

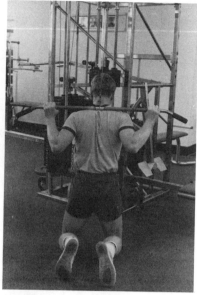

Contracted position

Muscles trained: latissimus dorsi

Grab the lat bar with an overhand grip and kneel directly under the bar. Pull the bar down to the base of the neck, pause and return to the starting position.

Key points:

- Keep the body vertical throughout the exercise.
- A spotter may be needed to hold the lifter down.

Bench press

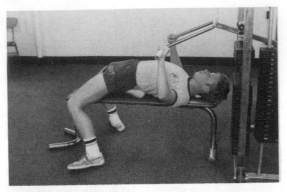

Starting position

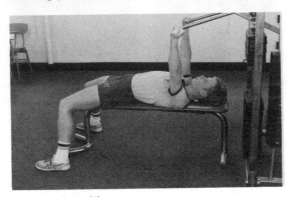

Extended position

Muscles trained: pectorals, deltoid, triceps

Lie on bench face up with chest directly under the bar. Knees are bent with feet flat on the floor. Keep the shoulders, back and buttocks in contact with the bench and press the weight to the extended position.

Key points:

- Shoulders, back and buttocks should be in contact with bench at all times.
- Do not push with the legs.
- Avoid resting in the extended position.

Seated press

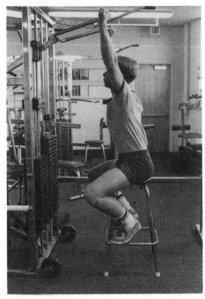 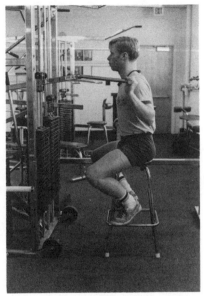

Starting position   **Extended position**

Muscles trained: deltoid, triceps

Seated at press station, shoulders should be directly under the bar with feet hooked on stool. Raise weight to the extended position and lower.

Key points:

- Do not arch back throughout lift.
- Maintain a vertical body position; avoid leaning.

Biceps curl

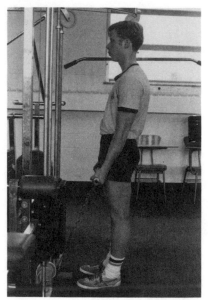 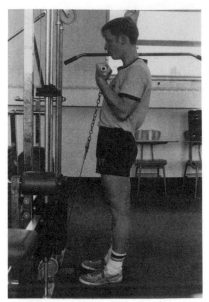

Starting position   **Contracted position**

Muscles trained: biceps

Hold curl bar in underhand grip with arms in the extended position. Keeping the upper arm stationary, raise weight to the contracted position, pause and lower to starting position.

Key points:

- Do not lean backward to facilitate lift.
- Hold elbows at sides; do not let them shift forward.

Triceps extension

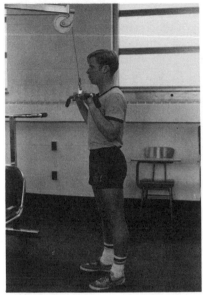 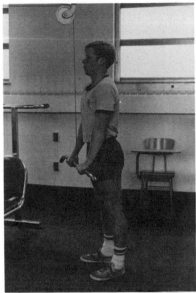

Starting position   **Extended position**

Muscles trained: triceps

Hold lat bar with a narrow overhand grip. Bend elbows and lift bar to the neck, keeping the upper arms and elbows fixed at sides. Moving only the lower arm, extend arms downward, pause and return to the starting position.

Key points:

- Keep elbows fixed at sides throughout lift.
- Avoid leaning forward.

Wrist curl

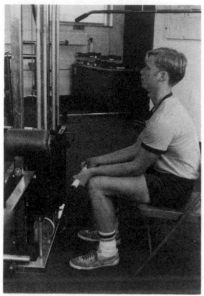 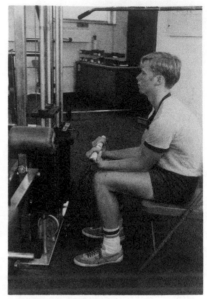

Starting position   **Contracted position**

Muscles trained: forearm flexors

Seated on chair facing curl bar, place forearms upon thighs with wrists extending past knees. Raise weight to the contracted position, pause and return to the extended position.

Key points:

- Elbows and forearms should maintain contact with thighs through entire lift.
- Concentrate on full-range movement.

Sit-ups

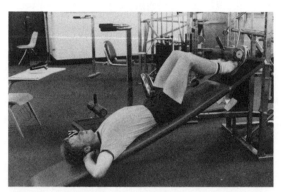

Starting position

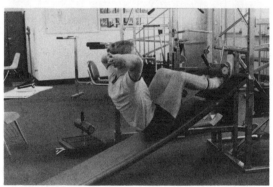

Contracted position

Muscles trained: abdominals

Adjust sit-up board according to level of fitness. Lie on back with feet locked in pads and knees bent. Interlace fingers behind the head. Keeping back curved, sit up to the contracted position and lower back to start.

Key points:

- Do not pull with the arms.
- Keep back curved throughout sit-up.
- Sit up on a two count and lower on a four count.

THE NAUTILUS MACHINES

Arthur Jones designed and marketed the Nautilus machine, so named because of the spiral pulley design of his first weight machine. It reminded him of the chambered nautilus, a mollusk of perfect geometric proportions.

It is precisely these pulleys and cams which enable an individual to train through the full range of motion; with variable resistance to the muscles throughout the exercise executed. Although the Nautilus machine may appear to be similar in appearance to a medieval torture machine, it becomes quite familiar as training progresses through the weeks and months.

Midshipmen enjoy working out on Nautilus machines. It is constantly necessary to stress, however, while the Nautilus machines are certainly excellent for developing muscular strength, they are by no means the only or best way to do it. All weight trainers must be constantly reminded that the key to success in training is correct application of all training principles, and this is equally true when training with Nautilus machines. The training principles, as outlined by the Nautilus Company, are shown below.

Nautilus training principles

General procedures to be followed in all machines where the regular (positive-negative) form of exercise is performed:

1. On any machine where seat adjustments or body positioning can be varied, make certain that the rotational axis of the cam is directly parallel to the rotational axis (joint) of the body part that is being moved.
2. Position your body in a straightly–aligned manner. Avoid twisting or shifting your weight during the movement.
3. Never squeeze hand grips tightly, but maintain a loose, comfortable grip (a tight squeeze elevates blood pressure).
4. Lift the resistance (positive work) to the count of two ... pause ... lower the resistance (negative work) slowly and smoothly while counting to four.
5. For full-range strength and flexibility (and protection against injury) your range of movement on each machine should be as great as possible.
6. Breathe normally. Try not to hold your breath while straining.

7. Perform each exercise for 8 to 12 repetitions.
    a. Begin with a weight you can comfortably do 8 times.
    b. Stay with that weight until you can perform 12 strict repetitions. On the following workout, increase the weight (approximately 5%) and go back to 8 repetitions.
    c. Ideally, on every workout you should progress in repetitions and/or resistance.
8. For best cardiorespiratory (heart-lungs) conditioning, move quickly from machine to machine (this speed does not apply to the actual exercises). The longer the rest between machines, the less effective the cardiorespiratory conditioning.
9. When possible, follow your routine as the exercises are numbered on your workout sheet; however, any time the machine you are to do next is being used, go to another exercise and then return to the machine that was in use.
10. All compound and double machines were designed to make use of the pre-exhaustion principle (where a single-joint exercise is used to pre-exhaust a given muscle and a multiple-joint exercise is used to force the exhausted muscle to work even harder); therefore, it is important to move very quickly (in less than 3 seconds) from the primary exercise to the secondary exercise.
11. Your training session should include a maximum of 12 exercises, 4 to 6 for the lower body and 6 to 8 for the upper body (a compound machine counts as two exercises).
12. Exercise the larger muscle groups first and proceed down to the smaller muscle groups (hips, thighs, back, shoulders, chest, arms, and neck).
13. Your entire workout should take from 20 to 30 minutes.
14. The time lapse between exercise sessions should be at least 48 hours and not more than 96 hours.

Training with Nautilus machines

When midshipmen request that a Nautilus training program be designed, the following steps are taken:

a.) Midshipmen are to become familiar with strength training principles, as discussed in this chapter.

b.) Midshipmen are to become familiar with the Nautilus training principles outlined on the previous page.

c.) Midshipmen are to become familiar with the record sheet listed below. The procedure is quite similar.

d.) Midshipmen are encouraged to begin their initial Nautilus training by carrying out the exercises indicated below.

Name _____

Date _____

Workout _____

Exercise	number						
Hip & Back	1						
Leg Extension	2						
Leg Press							
Leg Curl	3						
Double Chest	4a						
Pullover	5						
Torso Arm							
Lat Pulldown							
Lateral Raise	6a						
Seated Press	6b						
Shrugs							
Biceps	7						
Triceps Extension	8						
Calf Raisers	9						

The Nautilus machines and the listed exercises are shown, explained and discussed in the following pages.

Hip and back machine

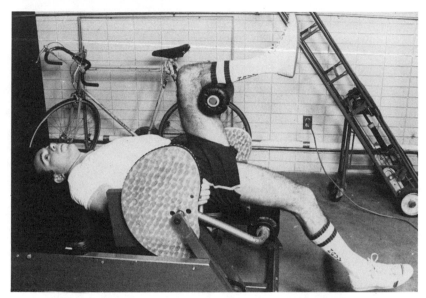

(Buttocks and lower back)

1. Enter machine from front by separating movement arms.
2. Lie on back with both legs over roller pads.
3. Align hip joints with axes of cams.
4. Fasten seat belt and grasp handles lightly.
5. Seat belt should be snug, but not too tight, as back must be arched at completion of movement.
6. From bent-legged position, extend both legs and at same time push back with hands.
7. Holding one leg at full extension, allow other leg to bend and come back as far as possible.
8. Stretch.
9. Push out until it joins other leg at extension.
10. Pause, arch lower back, and contract buttocks.
11. Repeat with other leg.

Important: In contracted position, keep legs straight, knees together, and toes pointed.

Leg extension machine

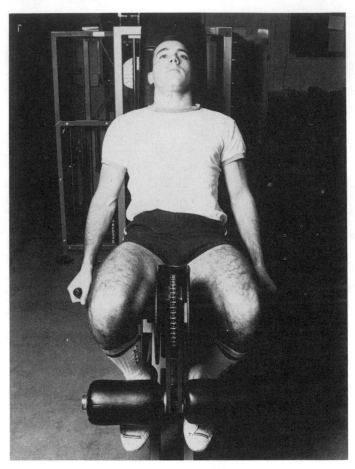

(Frontal thighs or quadriceps)

1. In a seated position, place feet behind roller pads with knees snug against seat.
2. Keep head and shoulders against seat back.
3. Straighten both legs smoothly.
4. Pause.
5. Slowly lower resistance and repeat.

Important: Avoid gripping handles tightly and do not grit teeth or tense neck or face muscles during movement.

Leg curl machine

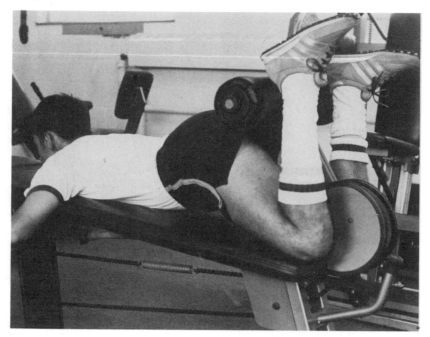

(Hamstrings)

1. Lie face down on machine.
2. Place feet under roller pads with knees just over edge of bench.
3. Lightly grasp handles to keep body from moving.
4. Curl lower legs and try to touch heels to buttocks.
5. When lower legs are perpendicular to bench, lift buttocks to increase movement.
6. Pause at point of full muscular contraction.
7. Slowly lower resistance and repeat.

Important: Top of foot should be flexed toward knee throughout movement.

Super pullover machine

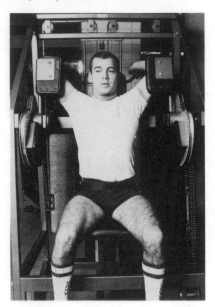 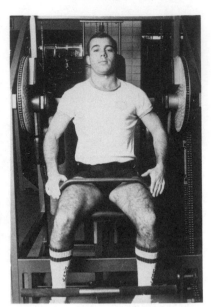

Pullover
(Latissimus dorsi muscles of the back and other torso muscles)

1. Adjust seat so shoulder joints are in line with axes of cams.
2. Assume erect position and fasten seat belt tightly.
3. Leg press foot pedal until elbow pads are about chin level.
4. Place elbows on pads.
5. Hands should be open and resting on curved portion of bar.
6. Remove legs from pedal and slowly rotate elbows as far back as possible.
7. Stretch.
8. Rotate elbows down until bar touches stomach.
9. Pause.
10. Slowly return to stretched position and repeat.
11. After final repetition, immediately do pulldown.

Important: Look straight ahead during movement. Do not move head or torso. Do not grip tightly with hands.

Double chest machine

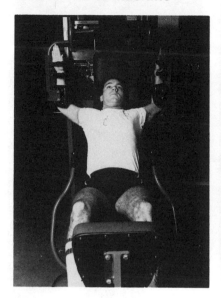 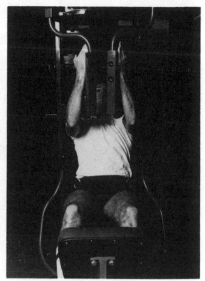

Arm cross
(Pectoralis majors of the chest and deltoids of shoulders)

1. Adjust seat until shoulders (when elbows are together) are directly under axes of overhead cams.
2. Fasten seat belt.
3. Place forearms behind and firmly against movement arm pads.
4. Lightly grasp handles (thumb should be around handle) and keep head against seat back.
5. Push with forearms and try to touch elbows together in front of chest. (Movement can also be done one arm at a time in an alternate fashion.)
6. Stretch at bottom and repeat pressing movement.
7. Slowly lower resistance and repeat.
8. After final repetition, immediately do decline press.

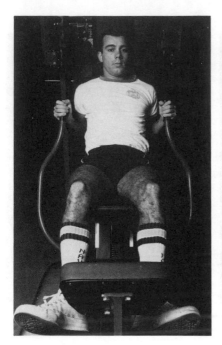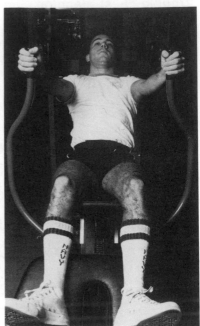

Decline press
(Chest, shoulders, and triceps of arms)

1. Use foot pedal to raise handles into starting position.
2. Grasp handles with parallel grip.
3. Keep head back and torso erect.
4. Press bars forward in controlled fashion.
5. Slowly lower resistance keeping elbows wide.
6. Stretch at point of full extension and repeat pressing movement.

Double shoulder machine

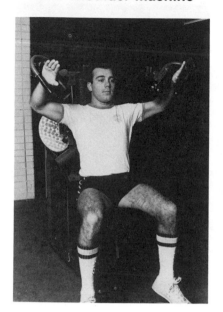 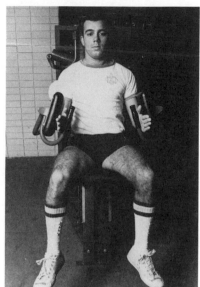

Lateral raise
(Deltoid muscles of shoulders)

1. Adjust seat so shoulder joints are in line with axes of cams.
2. Fasten seat belt.
3. Pull handles back until knuckles touch pads.
4. Lead with elbows and raise both arms until parallel with floor.
5. Pause.
6. Slowly lower resistance and repeat.
7. After final repetition, immediately do overhead press.

Important: Keep knuckles against pads and elbows high at all times.

Double shoulder machine

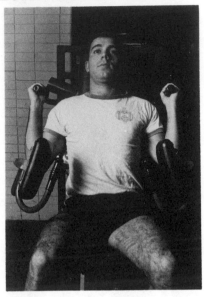 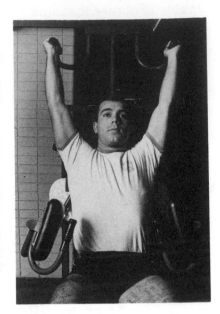

Overhead press
(Deltoids and triceps)

1. Grasp handles above shoulders.
2. Press handles overhead.
3. Slowly lower resistance, keeping elbows wide, and
   repeat.

Important: Do not arch back. Legs should be resting on seat
throughout both exercises.

Biceps/triceps machine

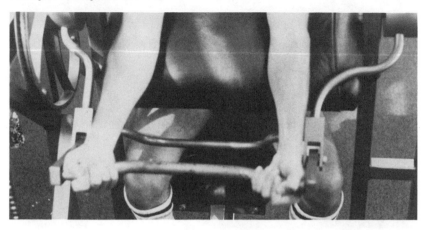

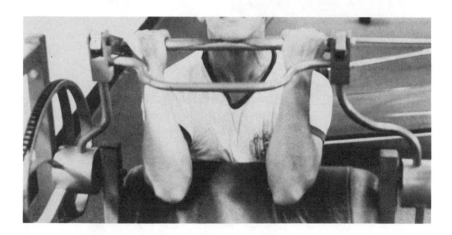

Biceps curl
(Biceps of upper arms)

1. Enter machine from left side.
2. Place elbows on pad and in line with axis of cam.
3. Grasp bar with palms up.
4. Smoothly curl bar until it reaches neck.
5. Pause.
6. Slowly return to stretched position and repeat.

Important: Lean back at full extension to insure stretching.

Biceps/triceps machine

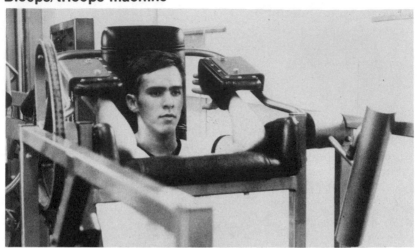

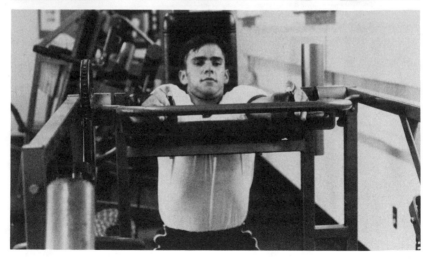

Triceps extension
(Triceps of upper arms)

1. Adjust seated position (with pads if necessary) until shoulders are on same level as elbows.
2. Place elbows in line with axis of cam and hands (with thumbs up) on pads.
3. Straighten arms smoothly.
4. Pause.
5. Slowly return to stretched position and repeat.

Multi-exercise machine

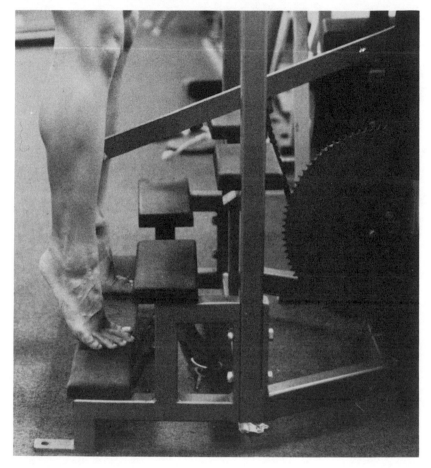

Calf Raises
(Calves)

1. Adjust belt comfortably around hips.
2. Place balls of feet on first step and hands on third step.
3. Lock knees and keep locked throughout movement.
4. Elevate heels as high as possible and try to stand on big toes.
5. Pause.
6. Slowly lower your heels.
7. Stretch at bottom by lifting toes.
8. Repeat.

RESULTS OF MUSCULAR FITNESS TRAINING

Physical benefits

After a six-week training period, those who have trained correctly with weights—be it free weights, the Universal Gym or Nautilus machines—will notice an improved appearance, because the muscles are firmer, larger and more efficient. Such strength efficiency is important in carrying out our daily assigned tasks.

At the Naval Academy all midshipmen must meet minimum standards in physical education, particularly in the areas of muscular strength and endurance, and some midshipmen are unable to meet these requirements until an intensive six-week training period has taken place.

But muscular fitness training can have benefits for everyone: The homemaker who has begun to train with weights correctly will suddenly discover after a six-week period that miraculous events are taking place. Suddenly the heavy laundry basket begins to be lighter; heavy grocery bags can be handled with greater ease. Young mothers who are training may wonder why their infants do not seem to be getting heavier when they are lifting them during daily activities. These examples illustrate how gains in strength can enable individuals to carry out their daily activities with greater ease.

Psychological benefits

There can be no question about it. We feel better if we look better. If we look better, we gain self-respect. Others clearly sense how we feel about ourselves and react accordingly. As we gain in physical strength and as our appearance improves, we feel more at peace with ourselves and the world.

REFERENCES

1. Aamold, Walter. *Navy-Penn State Football Program* (Naval Academy Athletics, 1845-1945), p. 26.

2. Brown, C., and J. Wilmore. "Effects of Maximal Resistance Training on the Strength and Body Composition of Women Athletes.", *Med. Sci. Sports,* Vol. 6, p. 171, 1974.

3. Cox, Jay S., and Heinz W. Lenz. "Women in Sports: The Naval Academy Experience," *The American Journal of Sports Medicine,* Vol. 7, No. 6, 1979.

4. Darden, Ellington. *Strength Training Principles: How to Get the Most Out of Your Workouts.* Winter Park, Florida: Anna Publishing Co., Inc., 1977.

5. Mayhew, J., and P. Cross. "Body Composition Changes in Young Women With High Resistance Weight Traning,", *Research Quarterly,* Vol. 45, pp. 433-440, 1974.

6. Nautilus Sports/Medicine Industries. *Nautilus Instruction Manual.* Deland, Florida. (2nd Edition.)

7. Westcott, Wayne L. "Female Response to Weight Training,", *Journal for Physical Education,* Vol. 77, pp. 31-33, 1979.

8. Wilmore, J. "Alterations in Strength, Body Composition and Anthropometric Measurements Consequent to a 10 Week Weight Training Program,", *Med. Sci. Sports,* Vol. 6, pp. 133-138, 1974.

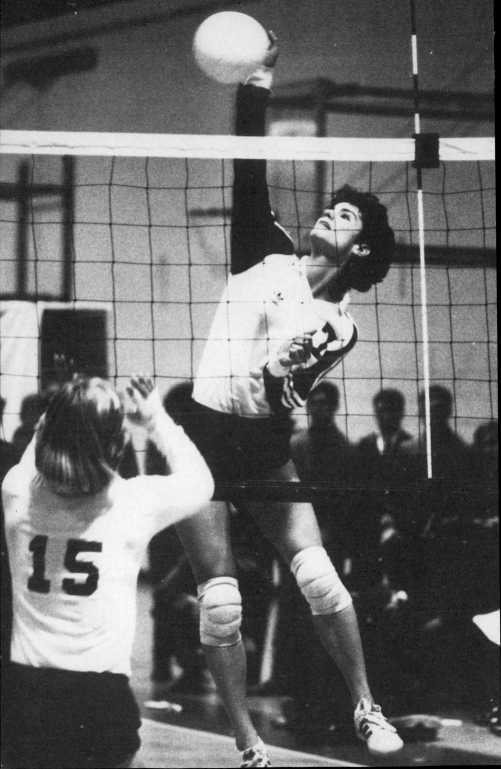

4

FLEXIBILITY FITNESS

The light grip made my arms soft so
my swing was smooth and easy . . .
the ball exploded off the club face.

Sam Snead

OBJECTIVES

- Define the term flexibility.
- List the main reasons why flexibility is important to the competitive athlete and non-competitive exerciser.
- Describe the most effective stretching technique.
- Identify several general exercises which are designed to improve the flexibility of various body segments.
- Illustrate the desired flexibility training methods for selected individual sports and exercise activities.
- List some of the precautions that should be taken when training to improve flexibility.

WHAT IS FLEXIBILITY?

Each of us has marvelled at the apparently effortless and graceful movements of the ice skater, the dancer, the gymnast and the acrobat. Their bodies seem to be "supple" despite the muscular power and endurance required to perform complex movements. These fluid-like and rhythmical movements are possible because of the athlete's high degree of flexibility.

Except for exercise and sports activities such as gymnastics, dance, yoga and ice skating, flexibility training until recently was usually given secondary consideration. Only during brief warmup periods was there time devoted to the development and maintenance of flexibility.

Now, fortunately athletes and exercisers are beginning to view flexibility training as an equal and integral part of fitness and athletic training.

Flexibility Beaulieu defines flexibility as "the possible range of motion or movement of a particular joint or group of joints."[1] Flexibility fitness therefore refers to the extent to which a full range of movement can occur at specific joints or in combinations of joints throughout the body. From the aspect of application, flexibility is the degree to which an individual can reduce muscle tension and stretch connective tissue around joints while performing sports and exercise activities. Beaulieu further states: "Because flexibility is not a general body factor but is specific to each individual joint or group of joints, it would seem inappropriate to label one person more flexible than another."[2]

TESTS OF FLEXIBILITY

Genetic factor Doug Morton,[3] Physiotherapist from the Denver Sports Medical Clinic, who has extensive experience with football players, indicates that some athletes are naturally "tight" and others are "loose." Morton stated that the muscle-tight athlete needs to work on flexibility but the muscle-joint-loose athlete probably needs more weight training. Five simple tests that determine whether an athlete is tight or loose follow:

1) Elbow Hyperextension—The athlete extends his arms to see if both elbows overextend (bend backwards at the joint).
2) Hip Laxity—The athlete, in a standing position, touches the backs of his heels together so that his feet point in opposite directions.
3) "Back-Knee" Extension—The athlete stands erect. If the knees overextend this is a sign of looseness.
4) Toe Touching—The athlete bends over and touches his toes without bending the knees. This tests for loose back and hamstring muscles.
5) Palms up, Palms down—The athlete extends his arms in front, turning the palms up. If the palms rotate beyond 180 degrees, this is a sign of laxity.

Beaulieu[4] suggests a more systematic and comprehensive approach to estimating the degree of flexibility. Throughout his text he illustrates a pre-screening test for each major movement of the body. Since flexibility is joint-specific, these tests help an individual determine where in the body to concentrate training.

Trunk flexion and extension Two of the more common general measures of flexibility are trunk flexion and trunk hyperextension. They are perhaps the most widely used tests because flexibility of the lower back or torso is directly affected in most exercise and sports activities. There is also a general interest in these tests because chronic lower backache is a major physical ailment for many individuals.

Lower-back problems are the number-one ailment affecting middle-aged and older adults. Although many theories abound regarding the causes of backaches, they are partly caused by a gradual loss of lower torso flexibility (mainly from disuse and inactivity among adults). Additional contributing factors are 1) the increased amount of body fat which accumulates around the abdominal and hip areas as people age (this of course is not a natural phenomenon—it results from overeating and under-exercising); and 2) the loss of muscle strength (tone) of the abdominal and lower spinal support muscles.

The trunk flexion and hyperextension tests are easily administered and are illustrated below:

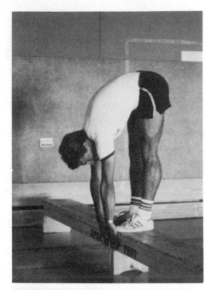 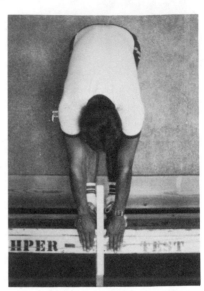

Trunk Flexion

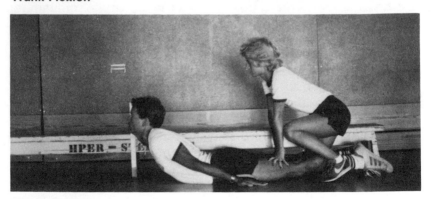

Trunk Extension

Trunk flexion

The trunk flexion test measures the degree of flexibility in the posterior back and spine muscles and the hamstring muscles when the legs are extended. Average flexibility of these combined groups would enable you to reach your toes with your fingertips. Reaching beyond the toes indicates better than average flexibility, and not reaching your toes indicates below average. Females generally should average one to two inches more reach than males.

Trunk extension

The trunk extension (hyperextension) test assesses the degree of flexibility of the anterior trunk and spine muscles in tandem with the quadriceps. Have a partner hold your legs and buttocks down as you lift your upper body with your hands locked behind your neck. Measure the distance in inches from the floor to your chin with a fixed ruler, or have an assistant holding a ruler do it. Average scores for females are 15-18 inches and for males 18-21 inches.

WHY FLEXIBILITY TRAINING?

In addition to achieving the desired dynamic movement patterns required in specific activities, there are other well-established reasons to engage in regular flexibility training. Perhaps the two main reasons for such training are expressed by Bob Anderson.[5] He states that when athletes have stretched regularly and correctly it helps them avoid injuries and perform to the best of their abilities.

In the same article Anderson indicates that stretching (the name given to the action which develops flexibility) as part of your daily activities will help you do the following:[6]

- Reduce muscle tension and help the body feel more relaxed.
- Improve coordination by allowing for freer and easier movement.
- Increase range of motion.
- Prevent injuries such as muscle strains.
- Make strenuous activities like running easier because it prepares you for the stress; it is a way of signaling the muscles that they are about to be used.
- Develop body awareness.
- Promote circulation.

Beaulieu[7] has conducted an extensive review of most of the scientific literature about flexibility. He also offers the most objective analysis of how flexibility training affects other parameters of physical performance. Several of the more important ones will be presented.

Prevention of muscle soreness and injury Competitive athletes and non-competitive athletes have at some point in their life experienced muscular soreness and muscular stiffness. Whenever we engage in unique physical movements requiring exertion above our normal or trained levels, we may experience such pains in our muscular system. Soreness and injury may result from sports participation, recreational pursuits and certain occupational tasks. Soreness and injury usually result when our muscles are used improperly, or out of balance with other muscles, for extended periods.

By designing a good flexibility fitness program, we can often reduce the degree of severity if soreness or injury do occur. Many professional athletic teams are discovering significant reductions of soft tissue injuries following the initiation of an appropriate flexibility program.

Speed, agility and strength In addition to the prevention of costly injuries (which sometimes motivate an athlete to do more flexibility exercises regularly), performance benefits may also result from flexibility training.

An individual athlete may accumulate benefits associated with the skill components of fitness, including agility, speed, coordination and reaction time. Although research is not exactly clear about specific benefits, studies have shown that better performers in swimming, gymnastics and other sports often have greater flexibility than their poorer-performing colleagues. Studies reported by Beaulieu also indicate that if a performer combines strength training with flexibility training, greater speed results than with strength or flexibility training alone.

The more flexible one is, the less fatigue one experiences in repetitive movements. One need only observe the unskilled, inflexible and fatiguing efforts of a poor swimmer when compared to the proficient swimmer. In this instance skill and flexibility combine to produce an efficient low-energy-expending movement.

Psychological benefits Although not extensively researched, flexibility training also produces some psychological side benefits. Athletes and older exercisers report overall general relaxation plus more freedom of movement following flexibility exercises.

These "good" feelings more than likely have a physiological basis. This physiological basis may include improved circulation and oxygen distribution through the soft tissue, the reduction of muscle tension from the act of stretching, the lubrication of the joints with synovial fluid and an increase in tissue temperature.

Psychologically, athletes who have high levels of flexibility also are confident in performing all-out effort without the fear of injury. Deconditioned and unskilled individuals with poor flexibility often express concern about possible injury during activity. Fortunately this assumption is usually correct, thus indicating the need for flexibility training. The fear of injury usually produces unwarranted tension in muscles. The reduction of concern for injury therefore allows the athlete to reduce muscular tension which improves reaction time and speed. This reduced muscle tension results in better performance.

Long-range benefits Although there have not been extensive studies to determine the effects of flexibility training on the muscle system of older individuals, it is clear that the slowed movements of the aged are due in part to the lack of flexibility. Accidents among the aging are indirectly the result of the inability of muscles, tendons and ligaments to stretch adequately. Perhaps one of the keys to an active and vigorous old age is daily flexibility training. As senior citizens become more active (and there is evidence that more and more of them are becoming physically active), more will be learned about the flexibility of aging tissue.

STRETCHING FOR FLEXIBILITY FITNESS

The word "flexible," according to Webster's New World Dictionary, means, "able to bend without breaking; pliant."[8] When used in the exercise context, flexibility refers to the ability to bend the joints of the body fully without injuring them.

A word often used interchangeably with flexibility is "stretching." The same Webster's dictionary defines *stretch* as, "to reach out to full length."[9] In practical terms, stretching refers to the act of elongating muscle and other soft tissue around joints during movement.

The most effective way to improve flexibility fitness is by engaging in "stretching" exercises. Muscles that have lost their flexibility because of disuse or improper use must be gradually and progressively stretched (elongated). Also, because many of our sports activities tend to enhance and reduce the range of movement in different body joints, simultaneously, we often need to supplement our sports involvement with stretching exercises.

Aside from the flexibility developed through various sports and exercise activities, specific stretching exercises may be performed. When muscles have been inactive for a period of time, effective stretching exercises should consist of static and rhythmic stretching rather than the formerly-used ballistic type of stretching.

Static stretching These exercises refer to placing the muscles on a full stretch and holding that position for ten (10) to thirty (30) seconds. It is recommended that you consciously attempt to release the tension from the fully-stretched muscle group, which will permit further stretching and add to your progressive stretching program.

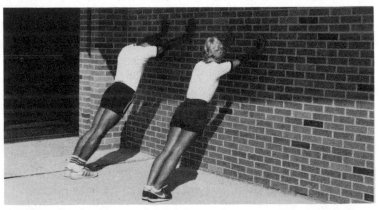

Calf Stretch

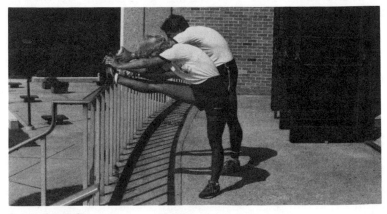

Groin Stretch

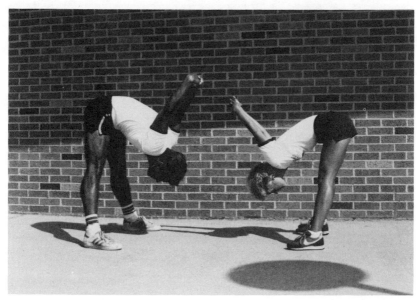

Shoulder Girdle Stretch

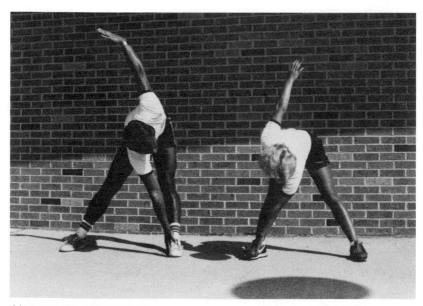

Alternate Trunk Stretch

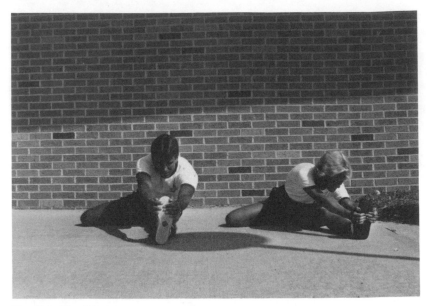

Hurdler Stretch

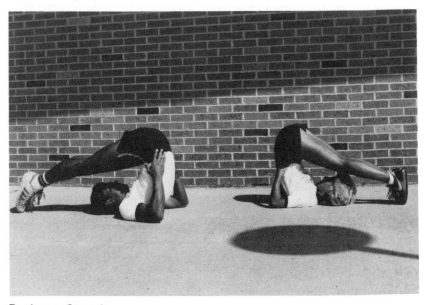

Backover Stretch

Ballistic stretching This term refers to the repetitive "bouncing" or "jerking" movements commonly seen among exercisers. This type of exercise is *not* recommended because it tends to stimulate the body's natural injury defense system—the stretching or muscle tendon reflex. Rapid stretching of a muscle produces this reflex, which is designed to prevent the muscle from being injured during overstretch. Rapid bouncing movements performed against a fully-stretched muscle tend to elicit this response and cause injury or severe muscle soreness.

Rhythmic stretching Following a period of slow static stretching you may wish to perform a series of slow rhythmical exercises such as arm or leg circles, alternate toe touches or jumping jacks prior to engaging in more vigorous exercise or sport activity. The transition from static to vigorous exercise through rhythmic exercises will also assist in gradually increasing your heart rate, elevating your body temperature and promoting greater blood circulation through your muscles.

When performed at full joint range, these exercises contribute to flexibility fitness and improvement in muscular fitness. Rhythmic stretching exercises should not be confused with ballistic stretching. Unlike ballistic exercises, which involve direct force against the joint with abrupt changes in direction, rhythmic movements are more continuous and of a rotary nature without rapid direction changes.

Stretching routine There are perhaps hundreds of ways to stretch different muscles from various postures. Individual preferences (and precautions) should determine the best routine for you. One possible routine is to begin with the head/neck area and work through the various muscle groups down to your feet and toes. You might prefer to work the opposite way from toes to the head and neck. Another popular option is to work on exercises in the standing position, then in the kneeling position, followed by the sitting and lying positions. Whatever routine of exercises you choose it should systematically flow from one exercise to the other. Keep in mind also that from time to time you may wish to change the routine. Having several routines to choose from keeps boredom out of your flexibility program.

When to perform flexibility exercises Training for flexibility can be done separately or in conjunction with other exercise. Some individuals prefer to stretch just after waking up in the morning.

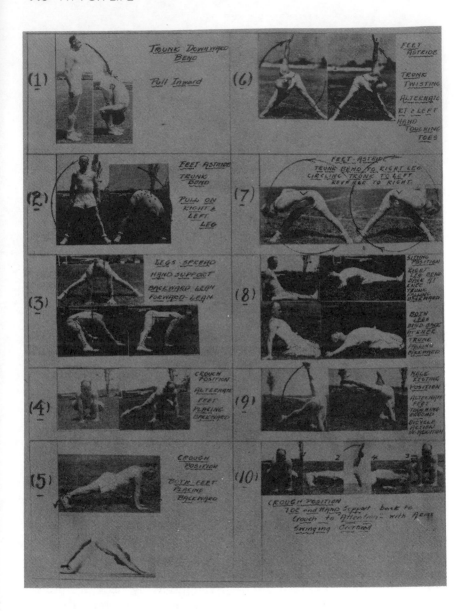

Flexibility and stretching exercises by Tommy Taylor.
(USNA historical photograph)

This helps them become more alert by stimulating circulation through the muscles. Psychologically it puts them in a positive mood for the day's activities.

Other people prefer to do flexibility exercises prior to more vigorous exercise. They serve as a warmup to more strenuous activity and also promote flexibility improvement. Others include flexibility training in their regular workout. Arthur Jones,[10] founder of the Nautilus system, argues effectively that proper use of the Nautilus equipment is the best way to develop strength and flexibility simultaneously.

Stretching *after* vigorous exercise is also recommended as a means to prevent muscular soreness. In fact, many exercise authorities now subscribe to the theory that it is more important to stretch *after* rather than *before* strenuous activity.

In general, however, individual preference and scheduling at your own convenience should determine when and how you train for flexibility. The important reminder is that flexibility should be considered an important element in your fitness program.

FLEXIBILITY FOR GENERAL FITNESS

Individuals who are primarily interested in maintaining a high level of general fitness should consider a program which improves or maintains flexibility throughout the body. Those who enjoy participating in a variety of sports and fitness-stimulating activities should also design a flexibility program to complement these activities. Persons who are more interested in a single sport or exercise are encouraged to develop general body flexibility. If this is not possible, they should particularly focus on joint movements which are directly related to their particular sport.

Clearly, anyone interested in fitness should have an understanding of the structure of the human body. By knowing what movements affect various muscle segments of the body, evaluating current levels of flexibility and designing a proper program are possible. Familiarize yourself with the anatomical illustrations in Chapter 3 and the possible ways in which you can move to improve flexibility of various muscle groups.

FLEXIBILITY TRAINING PROGRAMS

Training for flexibility may result from specific programs designed for that purpose or as an ancillary component of other sport or exercise activities. The following are some of the more general ways you can develop and maintain flexibility fitness.

Calisthenic activities Calisthenic-type activities conducted independently or as a warmup to a sports contest will promote flexibility fitness when conducted properly. Most of these exercises do not have sufficient resistance to improve muscular strength, nor are they repetitive enough to improve muscular endurance. Often the heart rate is not elevated to reach the aerobic training zone, and there is therefore no training effect to induce cardiovascular fitness. Because a benefit of calisthenics is flexibility, the participant should be sure that the exercises are performed in a manner which assures such results.

Music-guided activities Rhythmical calisthenic-type exercises choreographed in dance form to music are also excellent and fun ways to improve flexibility fitness. Popular programs such as aerobic dancing, jazz exercises and so on, can maximize flexibility development if the movements are performed at full range. Some of the movements essential to these programs however, may reduce the flexibility of certain muscle groups. Most of these programs do have supplemental stretching programs which easily compensate for these shortcomings, however.

An added benefit of these music-guided activities is the aerobic (cardiovascular) effect if performed according to the training principles. These programs truly are fun, sociable and satisfying ways to improve aerobic fitness.

Weight-training activities One might assume that because weight training tends to increase muscle mass, this form of training reduces flexibility. Upon close examination, just the opposite appears to be true. If weight-training exercises are performed through optimal full range of joint mobility, as is the case with much of the Nautilus equipment, these programs may be the best method to facilitate rapid flexibility development.

An individual's particular body build and muscular development may be somewhat deceiving with respect to the degree of flexibility present. For example, the muscular male gymnast must be extremely flexible to perform the complex movements required in that sport. On the other hand, the thin and apparently flexible-looking long-distance runner may be very inflexible in certain joints of the body as a result of that activity.

Sports activities As mentioned previously, participation in some sports activities may enhance or reduce flexibility. Furthermore, a given sport may enhance flexibility in certain body joints but decrease flexibility in other joints. For example, swimming may greatly improve the flexibility of the shoulder joint, shoulder girdle and ankle, but tighten the muscle groups around the knee and hip joints.

Most of us also experience an apparent loss of flexibility when we attempt to change from one sports activity to another. This is particularly evident when the sports involve different movement patterns. Sports activities in general, when selected carefully, can increase flexibility. To some extent the sports in which you participate should be selected on the basis of their flexibility component—especially if you are interested in improving total fitness through your sport.

Rehabilitative activities Flexibility is often lost following a period of inactivity caused by a physical impairment or injury. This reduction in mobility is caused by a loss of muscular fitness as well as flexibility.

Because flexibility reponds well to passive exercises (exercises performed by someone applying external force) this may be the preferred way to initially restore lost mobility. Resistance exercises may be added as full mobility is regained. In instances of severe disability, flexibility conditioning is appropriate and may provide the major stimulus toward improved tissue health.

Relaxation-promoting activities Exercises such as yoga, which are performed with minimum exertion but require proper training to achieve desirable results, also provide an excellent means to improve flexibility. For correct execution, these exercises additionally require the development of proprioceptive balance, muscular development that is balanced, and a relaxed mental state. The quieting of the mind prompts the release of muscular tension, thus enabling the individual to improve flexibility efficiently and effortlessly.

The huge payoff in these exercises, especially for the overly stressed individual, is the control and release of stress-producing muscular tension.

Flexibility circuit There are virtually unlimited ways to design a flexibility circuit program. Many of the current self-improvement magazines which often feature celebrities doing their favorite calisthenic-type exercises show many variations of the same themes. By combining any number of these different exercises, one can easily design a flexibility circuit which is personally appealing and at the same time beneficial. Another variation of the circuit is to combine flexibility training with muscular and/or aerobic fitness exercises. The possibilities are limited only by one's imagination and creativity.

FLEXIBILITY TRAINING PRECAUTIONS

Nearly everyone, including those with severe movement limitations, can benefit from flexibility training. Regardless of age, sex and present level of fitness, there are several precautions which should be adhered to when performing stretching exercises.

- Avoid stretching muscles to the point of intense pain. Attempt instead to stretch muscles to the point of maximum stretch, a point just below the threshold of pain.

- Avoid progressing too rapidly. Flexibility training should be a gradual process. Attempts to progress too fast often result in injuries and soreness.

- Avoid complex stretching movements initially. At first, stretch the major muscles of the body with simple, single-joint movements, then progress gradually to multiple-joint stretching.

- Avoid stretching one side of the body only or in one direction only. Always seek to train muscles of the body in balance with one another. Be sure to train both sides of the body equally. At a specific joint, both the agonist and antagonist muscle groups should be trained in balance.

- Avoid intense stretching that involves joints or muscles which are painfully sore or have recently been injured. Occasionally easy (light or nonresistive) stretching may help relieve *mild* muscle soreness.

- Avoid ballistic (bouncing, or jerky, rapid-change-of-direction) stretching. This may cause a stretch reflex and produce undesirable muscle soreness.

- Avoid participating in exercise and sport activities in a manner which causes stretching of muscle and soft tissue beyond your current flexibility level. For example, if you are deconditioned and decide that you want to play volleyball, you perhaps should play recreational (low intensity) volleyball for a period of time before suddenly engaging in highly competitive play.

DOWN THE STRETCH

Competitors and non-competitors in nearly every sport and exercise activity are now recognizing the importance of flexibility training as part of their personal fitness programs. Regular flexibility training can help prolong the career of the athlete and can help the exerciser enjoy active participation well into the later years of life.

As you construct your own fitness program, be certain that flexibility training is an integral part of that training.

REFERENCES

1. Beaulieu, John E., *Stretching for All Sports*. Pasadena, CA.: The Athletic Press, 1980, p. 13.
2. *Ibid.*, p. 13.
3. *Ibid.*, pp. 143-144.
4. *Ibid.*
5. Anderson, Bob, *The Runner*. September 1980, p. 24.
6. *Ibid.*, p. 24.
7. Beaulieu, John E., *Stretching for All Sports*. Pasadena, CA.: The Athletic Press, 1980.
8. Webster's *New World Dictionary*. New York: Simon and Schuster (second college edition), 1980.
9. *Ibid.*
10. Jones, Arthur, *Athletic Journal*. March 1977.

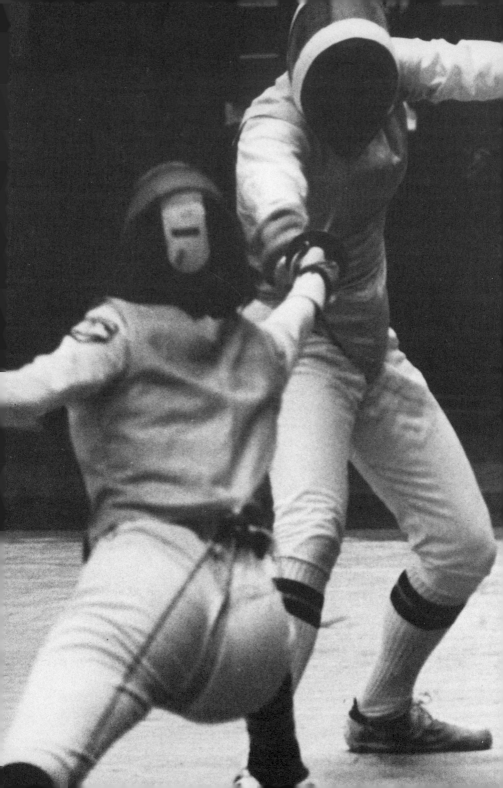

5

CIRCUIT TRAINING FOR TOTAL FITNESS

Athletic ability is a gift. Physical fitness is a reward.

—Capt. Jay Cox, MD, USN

OBJECTIVES

- Trace the beginnings of circuit training.
- Define circuit training.
- Give examples of exercises and circuits used by midshipmen at the Naval Academy.
- Examine recent findings in circuit training research.
- Distinguish between circuit and super-circuit training.
- Describe various super-circuit programs.
- Identify benefits resulting from circuit training.

WHAT IS CIRCUIT TRAINING?

In recent years circuit training has become a popular training method to achieve physical fitness. This training method is usually said to have begun at the University of Leeds, where exercises were presented, developed and put into practice in 1953 by R. E. Morgan and G. T. Adamson.[1] According to these two authors, circuit training has three major qualities:

1. It aims at the development of muscular and circulo-respiratory fitness.
2. It applies the principle of progressive overload (discussed in our text in Chapter 3, "Muscular Fitness").
3. It enables large numbers of performers to train at the same time by employing a circuit of consecutively numbered exercises around which each performer progresses, doing a prescribed allocation of work at each exercise, and checking progress against the clock.

These principles of exercise were known before Morgan and Adamson described circuit training, however.

In the early 1930s one of the authors of this text attended a small, private elementary school in Berlin, Germany. The school was housed in a private villa. Surrounding the villa was a strip of grass, approximately fifteen feet in width. Around this entire circumference, various types of gymnastic apparatus, ranging from parallel bars to balance beams to simple swings and lines attached to trees, were set up. Every morning before classes began, the entire student body of 70-80 boys and girls was divided into twenty groups (because there were twenty exercise stations surrounding the villa) so that there were three or four students at each of the stations. At the sound of a bell, all exercised at their station for thirty seconds; then the bell rang again and all progressed to the next station. At every fifth station boys and girls ran one lap around the villa. Within one-half hour all boys and girls had exercised at each of the stations and had run at least four times around the school.

Although this exercise period was not called circuit training, but simply "Die Turnstunde," it was what Morgan and Adamson would twenty years later write about.

Arrangements of stations An infinite variety of circuits is possible. An example of an excellent circuit is found in this text in Part III, Chapter 11, a circuit designed to fit on the small torpedo deck of a destroyer. It is evident that a circuit can be set up in a minimum of space. There are different methods of arranging circuits and distinction must be made between circuits based only on weight-training exercises and circuits which incorporate cardiovascular fitness training.

Traditional circuits In traditional circuits there might be eight stations, at each one of which a weight-training exercise is carried out. When all eight stations have been completed, individuals will have trained all major muscle groups.

Circuit training for high levels of fitness It is indeed possible to design a circuit for warming up, flexibility, muscular strength, cardiovascular fitness and most certainly for specific sports— circuits where specific skills are practiced. Many coaches and physical educators designed such circuits. Those who designed circuits for weight training, which in fact were simply a series of weight training exercises training all muscle groups, claimed that their circuit was best for total fitness. Those who designed circuits in which aerobic fitness was stressed were convinced that this type of training led to total fitness.

Total physical fitness In Chapter 1 our readers learned the meaning of physical fitness. It was explained that there are three primary components of physical fitness: cardiovascular fitness, muscular fitness and flexibility fitness. It is clear then that only those circuits which include stations or provisions to train all three primary components are effective for achieving total physical fitness. If a circuit includes only weight-training exercises, only muscular fitness will be achieved; if a circuit is designed so that the heart rate is maintained within the appropriate training zone (Chapter 2, Table 2), only aerobic fitness is achieved. The key to total fitness through circuit training is to design a circuit which includes all three primary components of physical fitness. Examples of two circuit training programs designed for midshipmen are described in the following pages.

CIRCUIT TRAINING
Program 1
The Universal Gym and Jogging Half-Miles

For record keeping, pounds to be lifted, and number of repetitions, consult Chapter 3.

1. The warmup
- Carry out the exercises described in Chapter 2.
- Jog one-half mile very slowly.

2. Chest press While lying on a bench on your back, grip the bar at shoulder width. Lower the bar to your chest, then explode the bar to arm's length. You may use a wide and a narrow grip along with medium grip for the three different sets. Inhale as the bar comes down, exhale as the bar goes up.

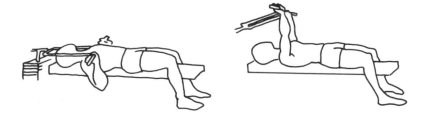

3. Leg press On Universal Gym, sitting in the leg press chair, begin with the knees toward the body. Explode the legs, extending the knee to full extension. Exhale at completion of the leg press, inhale coming back.

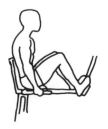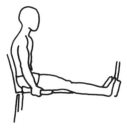

4. Shoulder press Using the Universal Gym, seat yourself at the shoulder press station. Start the press with the hands in front of the chest with body facing the machine. Explode the arms to full extension. Return to starting position. Inhale coming down, exhale at top going up.

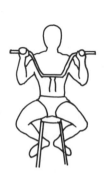 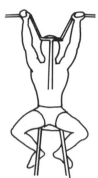

5. Jog one-half mile

6. Leg raises Lie on your back on a low bench with your head toward the rollers. Grasp the rollers with both hands. Keep your shoulders flat on the bench. Keeping the legs straight, pull them up as far as possible overhead, then lower them slowly to the flat position. Inhale while raising the legs, exhale while lowering. Repeat the exercise.

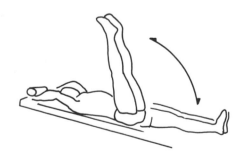

7. Lat pull-down On the Universal Gym from a kneeling position, grip the bar with arms fully extended. Pull the bar straight down in front of you as far as you can. Let the bar return to the starting position by giving way gradually against resistance. Breathe in going up and exhale coming down.

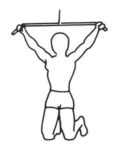 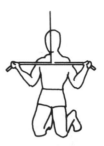

8. Calf raises Using the Universal Gym, adjust the chair to maximum distance from machine. Place the ball of your foot on the bottom edge of the pedal. Concentrate on complete extension of the toes. Explode. Breathe in going down, breathe out coming up.

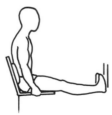 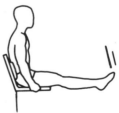

9. Upright rowing Stand erect facing machine. Narrow grip (handles together). Pull elbows high and hands under chin. Inhale up high in the chest. Exhale down. (Blow weight down.)

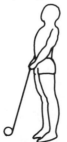 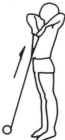

10. Double arm curl Stand erect, the body braced backward. Use a narrow grip with palms facing forward. Curl palms toward shoulders, bending elbows to bring bar in an arc to the chest. Inhale up, exhale down. (Blow weight down.)

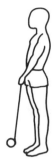 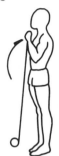

11. Jog one-half mile

12. Leg extension Sit erect with your insteps under the lower roller pads. Extend your legs until your knees lock out at horizontal position. Lower under control and repeat. Breathe in prior to extertion and blow out as extension occurs.

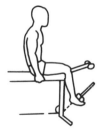 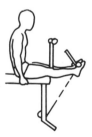

13. Leg curls Lie facing the weight stack with your heels placed under the top padded rollers. Raise up on your elbows and pull your heels toward your buttocks. Explode during this exercise and lower under control. Breathe in prior to exertion and exhale as you let the weight down.

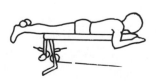 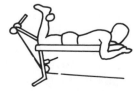

14. Bent -knee sit-ups (incline) Position yourself on an incline board with the head down, the knees fully bent, and the hands behind the head. Bend at the waist to an upright position and touch the left elbow to the right knee, the right elbow to the left knee and return to starting position.

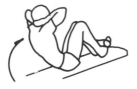 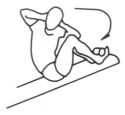

15. Cool down Walking five to ten minutes before going to the shower or bath.

This type of circuit training program is designed for midshipmen who are seeking an excellent level of physical fitness. It is estimated that the entire program takes from 40 to 45 minutes. The intensity of the program can be reduced or increased, depending on the pace set for the half-mile jog. In addition, it may be desirable to maintain the number of repetitions at eight or twelve, depending on the muscle group trained. (Consult Chapter 3, page 94)

Circuit Program 1
Variations

Cycling If it is practical and desirable, one may substitute cycling one and one-half miles instead of jogging one-half mile.
Swimming If swimming is desired instead of jogging, a distance of 220 yards may be substituted. It should be noted that the substitution of swimming creates practical problems, such as changing from a wet suit to dry clothing. However, such minor obstacles often do not prevent midshipmen from including swimming in their circuit training.

CIRCUIT TRAINING
Program 2
Nautilus Machines and Chair Stepping

For record keeping, pounds to be lifted, and number of repetitions, consult Chapter 3.

1. The Warmup • Same as for circuit training program 1.

2. Special Circuit Note: *Between each of the indicated stations step up and down a chair for sixty seconds, consult Chapter 2.

Name _____

Date _____

Workout _____

Exercise number

Hip *	1
Back	
Leg Extension	2
Leg Press	
Leg Curl	3
Double Chest	4a
Decline Press	4b
Pullover	5
Torso Arm	
Lat Pulldown	
Lateral Raise	6a
Seated Press	6b
Shrugs	
Biceps	7
Triceps Extension	8
Calf Raisers	

3. Cool down Walk five to ten minutes before going to the shower or bath.

This type of circuit training program is designed for midshipmen who desire to train in one location, rather than moving from one exercise area to another. Such a program is particularly desirable in case of inclement weather.

This particular program will unquestionably maintain high training heart rate because of the continued chair-stepping. Midshipmen are advised to interchange training stations if the next station in sequence is occupied. The key to circuit training is to maintain the heart in the appropriate training zone. The intensity of the program can be reduced or increased by the length of each chair-stepping exercise. In addition, just as in circuit program 1, the number of repetitions at each of the stations may be varied.

Circuit Program 2
Variations

- It is possible to apply the chair-stepping principle to circuit program 1.
- It is possible to apply the variations suggested in program 1 to program 2.

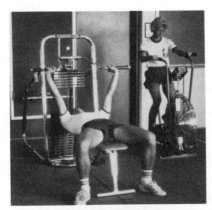

The Bench Press Station and The Exercise Bike

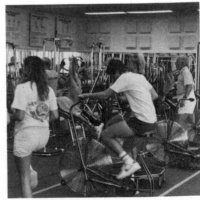

A View of the Supercircuit Circuit Training Area

RECENT FINDINGS IN CIRCUIT TRAINING

In Dallas, Texas, at the Institute for Aerobics Research, under the leadership of Research Director Larry Gettman, a significant contribution was made to circuit training.

The Research Institute reported that by incorporating running between exercise stations, caloric expenditure could be increased up to 27%, aerobic points could be doubled and up to 25% greater strength gains could be achieved than with regular circuit weight training.[3] These results were achieved by simply requiring that the exerciser run for 30 seconds between each exercise station. The Research Institute also reports that exercise bikes or indoor joggers, or both, may be substituted for the 30-second running portion. If weight lifting is combined with aerobic exercises in the same circuit, it is called "Super-Circuit" training, a term coined by the Universal Corporation.

Neither of the two circuit programs described above is, strictly speaking, a super-circuit. However, the principles are applied and the benefits are reaped.

A "Super-Circuit," in the truest sense of the word, is in operation at the Catonsville Community College, Catonsville, Maryland, where one of the authors helped with its design. Picture 1 makes it clear that adjacent to each weight training station is a station designed for aerobic fitness training. This station is either an exercise bike, or a station where jogging takes place, on a special piece of apparatus called an indoor jogger.

It can be seen that super-circuit training principles are similar to the principles described previously in this chapter.

Super-circuit training procedure
- Begin at any exercise station.
- Do not overexert; your pulse rate should remain within your training zone.
- Perform exercises through the full range of motion.
- Select a weight that allows you to perform 12-15 repetitions in a 30-second time period.
- Use a moderate weight 40-60% of maximum time lifting capacity at each station.
- At the end of 30 seconds (12 or 15 reps), the participant should immediately perform an aerobic exercise (running, exercise bike, rope skipping, trampoline) for 30 seconds.

- At the end of 30 seconds the participant proceeds immediately to the next exercise station without any rest intervals.
- The entire super-circuit is performed in a like manner, alternating 30 seconds of aerobic exercise with 30 seconds of weight training.
- The performer should concentrate on making the muscle contract explosively through the entire range of motion.
- Obviously, untrained persons should not attempt the super-circuit without a physical examination; they should be familiar with proper lifting technique and be progressively pre-conditioned to the stress of circuit training.

BENEFITS OF SUPER-CIRCUIT TRAINING

From the findings at the Dallas Aerobics Institute, it appears that super-circuit training provides benefits beyond those to be gained from ordinary circuit training.

- More calories were expended, and thus more weight was lost.
- A higher level of cardiovascular fitness was achieved because more liters of oxygen are used in the training.
- There is a distinct gain in muscular fitness.
- Provided varied training.

The fourth benefit is important and should be considered. Circuit training provides individuals with a great variety of activities, and the merits of variety in training for total physical fitness cannot be overemphasized.

A few years ago one of the authors had the following experience at the Naval Academy. He was contacted by an Academy graduate, a first lieutenant in the U.S. Marine Corps, who had the reputation of being a most conscientious and physically fit young man. The marine requested an appointment to discuss a physical fitness problem. During a meeting he related that around 11:00 A.M., as he started to think about his noon workout, he would begin to feel sick to his stomach; there were even times when he would have to leave his desk and vomit. Upon being questioned about his training, he told me what his training routine consisted of:

Warmup
- Jog an easy mile in 6 minutes and 30 seconds.
- Do 15 pull-ups.
- Do 3 flexibility exercises.
- Do 70 sit-ups in two minutes.

Running phase
- Run six one-half miles, each in 2 minutes and 30 seconds.

Strength phase
- Between each one-half mile do alternately 20 pull-ups or 85 sit-ups in two minutes.

Sprint phase
- Sprint 4, 6, or 8 times 60 yards.

The young marine officer had the routine neatly written down on a three-by-five index card enclosed in plastic. When questioned, he told me that he did his training every single day of the year, without missing a day, regardless of conditions. For four years he had trained precisely in this manner.

It was clear why this officer became sick when he thought about his training. We discussed at length the importance of not only varying the intensity of the workouts and the activities themselves, but also the importance of allowing the body to recover after a highly intensive workout by taking a day off from his training. We modified the program. The young man returned to me in four weeks. Not only had he introduced the required variety into his training, but he also had scored higher than ever in the quarterly Marine Physical Fitness Test.

Variety is essential in physical training, and circuit training lends itself to many varied physical activities. Progress will be made as long as our readers remember to stress the intensity, frequency and duration factors.

REFERENCES
1. Morgan, R.E. and G.T. Adamson, *Circuit Training*, London: G. Bell and Sons., Ltd., 1961.
2. Universal Gym Machines, *New Comprehensive Training Manual*. Irvine, CA: Universal Gym Equipment, 1978.
3. *The Winning Edge*, Vol. 1, No. 2, November-December 1980. Universal Gym, Cedar Rapids, IA.
4. Sorani, Robert, *Circuit Training*, Dubuque, IA: Wm. C. Brown Co., 1966.

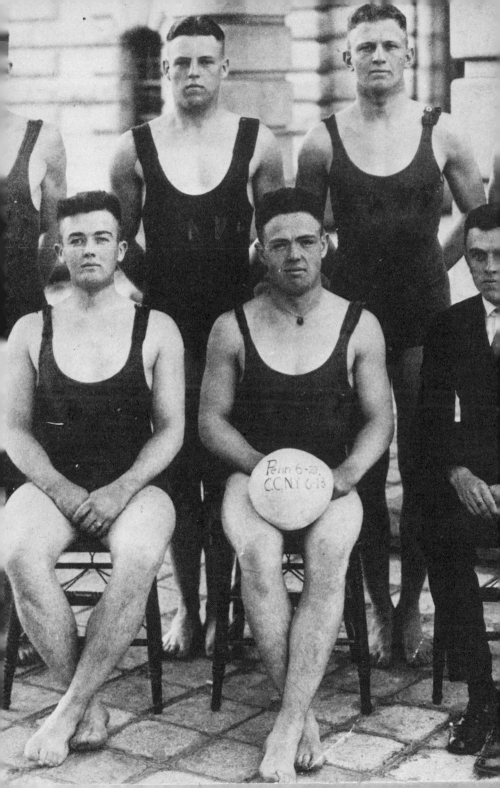

Penn 6-20.
C.C.N.Y. 6-13

PART II
FITNESS RELATED
HEALTH FACTORS

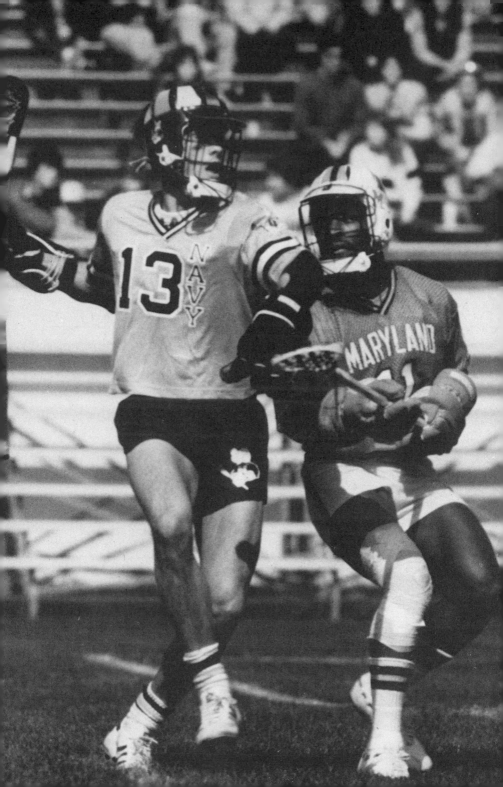

6

HEART DISEASE AND FITNESS

> You can no more give people health than you can give them wisdom. . . . learning and health are personal responsibilities.
>
> Dr. George Sheehan,
> *Sheehan on Running*

OBJECTIVES

- Identify the anatomical components of the human heart
- Describe the nervous and circulatory functions of the heart
- Compare current statistical rates of heart and blood vessel diseases
- Define atherosclerosis and explain how it underlies coronary heart and cerebral vascular diseases
- Identify the major risk factors associated with heart and blood vessel diseases
- Identify the most common methods of diagnosing cardiovascular disorders
- List several methods of treating heart disease
- Examine the role of exercise in cardiac rehabilitation
- Discuss the role of exercise in heart disease prevention and longevity.

INTRODUCTION

A book on physical fitness would not be complete without at least a brief description of the human heart and its associated functions. The serious student of fitness must clearly understand the relationship between muscular effort and its effect upon the cardiovascular system. It is only when the internal systems are stimulated according to selected training principles that fitness will result.

As the leading cause of death in the United States, diseases of the heart are another important subject for a fitness text. All of us need to identify and learn how to control heart disease risk factors. The heart patient is also vitally interested in whether exercise is beneficial or harmful.

We must expand our knowledge about heart disease. And we must take active measures to improve our fitness and help slow down this modern plague on human lives.

THE MIRACULOUS PUMP

Long before the anatomy and function of the heart were clearly understood, the organ was represented as having mystical and sacred qualities. The heart was the seat of the soul—the spiritual and emotional center of each person.

Despite our clearer understanding today of the heart's function, we often forget that it is an essential part of our physical body. Too often we ignore its needs and care about it only when something goes wrong. Still, even though we neglect this miraculous pump, it beats on well into seven, eight or nine decades of life. Perhaps we should take our automobile mechanic's advice about our car's engine and likewise begin a program of preventive maintenance before we have a major breakdown. Our lives may depend on it!

Heart structure

The human heart is not much larger than a clenched adult fist. It weighs less than a pound, but pumps over 20 tons of blood each day. With proper care it routinely beats over 100,000 times a day during an entire lifetime. Its force pushes blood to every cell of the body through a network of 60,000 miles of blood vessels.

The heart looks like an upside-down pear and lies beneath the protective breast bone, the sternum. It consists of four chambers. The right two chambers and the left two both form pumping units, and both function simultaneously as the two upper chambers (atria) pump blood into the two lower chambers (ventricles). The ventricles in turn pump harmoniously as the left ventricle pumps blood to the body via the aorta (the major artery leading from the heart), and the right ventricle pumps blood to the lungs through the pulmonary artery. A system of valves prevents blood backup. Two valves are located between the atria and ventricles, and two are located at the junction of the aorta and pulmonary arteries as they leave the heart.

Heart function

A sustained and regular heartbeat is maintained through counterbalancing nerve stimulation. This stimulation results from the parasympathetic system (vagus nerve) and the sympathetic system (accelerator nerve). Heart rate is also influenced by other factors, namely blood hormones such as epinephrine released during excitement by the adrenal glands.

Within the muscle tissue of the heart an intricate arrangement of nerve tissue and pathways give rhythm to the heartbeat. The muscular contractions of the atria respond to the stimulation of the sino-atrial node (SA node, or pacemaker) and the spread of electrical potential across the atrial membrane. This is followed closely by the signal being picked up by the atrioventricular node (AV node). This specialized nerve transmitter sends its powerful signal throughout the ventricles, causing them to contract forcefully. In modern medicine, the electrical activity of the heart can be observed through a diagnostic tool known as an electrocardiogram (EKG).[3]

Heart tissue and circulation The human heart is comprised of tough elastic connective tissue and uniquely-designed, specialized muscle tissue. The muscle tissue is formed by cells which are capable of beating independently. Each cell is a potential pacemaker, and together the cells can synchronize their activity into rhythmical contractions. The harmony of these cells is one of life's miracles.

Because of their unceasing working, heart muscle cells require a constant supply of nutrients and oxygen. This life-sustaining function results from blood supplied by the two main coronary blood vessels. Known as the left and right coronary arteries, their branches form a coronary (crownlike) tree throughout the heart. The arteries originate from the aorta at its

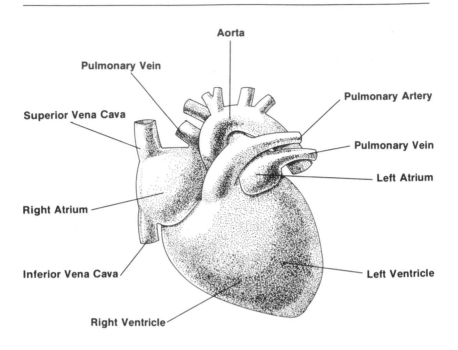

Aorta

Pulmonary Vein

Pulmonary Artery

Superior Vena Cava

Pulmonary Vein

Left Atrium

Right Atrium

Inferior Vena Cava

Left Ventricle

Right Ventricle

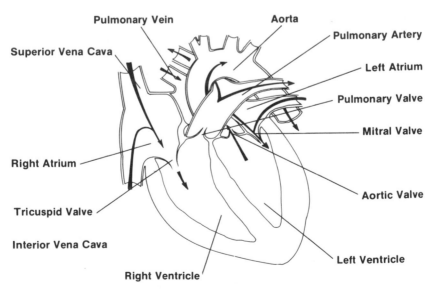

Pulmonary Vein

Aorta

Superior Vena Cava

Pulmonary Artery

Left Atrium

Pulmonary Valve

Mitral Valve

Right Atrium

Aortic Valve

Tricuspid Valve

Interior Vena Cava

Left Ventricle

Right Ventricle

junction with the heart. Blockages in one or more of these arterial branches cause one of today's major diseases—coronary heart disease.

La Machine

As you study the material in this chapter, remember that the human heart is a miraculous machine, a finely-tuned instrument designed to power your life's activities. You must treat it respectfully. Its ability to sustain your life and bring quality to your existence is your responsibility alone.

HEART DISEASE

In his autobiography, *My Life and Medicine*, the famous cardiologist Dr. Paul Dudley White wrote that heart disease began to be an epidemic in the 1940s and became a major one in the 1950s.[4] In the 1960s and 70s, over one million Americans annually died of heart and blood vessel diseases, and over sixty percent of those died of heart attacks. These one million deaths from heart and blood vessel diseases represent slightly over fifty percent of deaths from all causes in the United States. The prevalence of heart disease as a major crippler and killer in the United States had a significant impact upon the attitudes of many Americans toward health. Medical and educational programs were initiated in an attempt to end this epidemic of heart disease. Many programs focused attention on prevention.

One such effort was initiated by President Dwight Eisenhower in 1955. Prompted in part by his own heart attack and the negative results of a nationwide Kraus-Weber fitness test of fitness in American children, President Eisenhower created the President's Council on Physical Fitness. This Federal effort was directed at improving the health and fitness of American youth, which had performed poorly on a nationwide fitness test. Ike's cardiologist, Dr. Paul Dudley White, also received much notice at this time for his insistence that good lifestyle (diet and exercise) habits were the chief means of preventing heart disease.

In the early 1960s, President John F. Kennedy also had a significant impact on our efforts to improve our health as individuals and as a nation. His personal activities and his presidential proclamations regarding fitness stirred our health consciousness, as well as that of the Navy.

Research began to demonstrate a direct link between our affluent lifestyles and heart disease. Habits over which each of us had control, such as stress, smoking, proper diet, and amount of exercise, were being implicated as possible factors in heart disease.

Beginning in the 1960s and stretching on to the present day, Americans entered into a wellness revolution. Largely because of the messianic efforts of people like Dr. Kenneth Cooper, who published *Aerobics* in 1968,[6] the wave of health and fitness consciousness has spread to virtually every corner of America. From the innermost sectors of urban centers to the most remote villages, people are exercising, dieting and meditating their way toward improved personal health and fitness. Millions are discovering that they feel better physically, mentally and emotionally. They report a reduction in sickness and absenteeism from work. They have more vitality and energy, have reduced tensions (stress) and sleep better. For many, a return to increased interest in their physical bodies has also resulted in a renewed spiritual existence.

Decline in heart disease
At long last, there are indications that the epidemic of heart disease is on the decline. Statistics released by the National Institute of Health and other sources indicate a decrease of fatal heart disease ranging from three to five percent a year since the late 1960s.

As medical research and technology advance and individuals begin to take preventive health action—beginning in early childhood—heart disease will no longer be a significant health problem. The result will be healthier individuals to lead this country and the world into the super-technological age of humankind.

HEART DISEASE RISK FACTORS

Research efforts in the United States and throughout the world are fitting together the pieces of the heart disease puzzle. Although a number of contributory factors have been cited, many questions regarding the etiology of heart disease remain unanswered.

The search goes on to find definite answers to such questions as: How do risk factors interact to cause heart disease? What roles do heredity and environment play in causing the disease? Is heart disease predictable by analyzing risk factors? And can heart disease be prevented by changing, eliminating or controlling risk factors?

Persons interested in preventive health are not waiting for the detailed answers to these questions. Their personal experiences with friends and relatives who have died of heart disease and the current evidence is convincing enough. They have concluded that one's lifestyle is an important consideration in the development of heart disease. Millions of Americans have adopted healthier lifestyles—the tracks, bike paths, ski slopes, and gyms clearly reveal this dramatic change in attitude and behavior. However, too many other Americans remain sedentary, suffer from too much stress, smoke too much, overeat and become fat. This majority likely includes the cynical, the skeptical, the fatalists, the undisciplined (those who know better) and the unaware (those who do not know the facts). Perhaps a review of atherosclerosis and the risk factors once again will convince some of our friends to change their habits. Or a statement from one of the world's eminent physicians and foremost authorities on exercise physiology, Dr. Per-Olof Astrand, may be convincing.

In a special edition of the *Journal of Physical Education* in Summer of 1976 covering the Proceedings of the National YMCA Consultation on Cardiovascular Health, this authoritative Swedish researcher stated:

> Most of us consider that there is enough evidence to support the assumption that smoking, lack of exercise, rich foods and malnutrition are risks to health, even if the "evidence" is often rather circumstantial.[8]

Dr. Astrand further indicates that perhaps physicians must take a more active role in advising their patients about potential lifestyle risks. He wrote:

> I find it unfortunate, however, that so many physicians are applying a double standard when evaluating scientific evidence about the mentioned risk factors on the one hand, the more traditional therapeutic measures on the other. Any suspicion of harmful effects should have the same consequences in both cases. I repeat that physical inactivity gives rise to atrophy of certain tissues, to reduced cardiac function and increased fatigability.

There is hard evidence available on this point. I cannot explain why this evidence is not enough to arouse the whole-hearted interest of doctors in recommending recreational exercises.[9]

Atherosclerosis

A discussion of specific risk factors requires some knowledge of the underlying cause of heart disease. Atherosclerosis, the chief villain of blood vessel diseases, is a condition whereby arteries are narrowed by unwanted plaque formation on their interior walls. A slow, progressive condition believed to begin in childhood and prevalent mostly in the more technologically advanced countries, it can lead to fatal strokes and heart attacks. The condition becomes fatal if it progresses to the point of blocking major coronary or cerebral arteries, depriving them of vital nutrients and oxygen.

Several theories of atherosclerosis formation have been proposed. None clearly explains all clinical observations, however. Drs. Antonio Gotto and Michael Debakey, in their book, *The Living Heart*,[10] outline the crucial steps in the evolution of atherosclerotic lesions as follows:

1) damage to the endothelial lining
2) the focal accumulation of intimal lipids (fats)
3) the proliferation of the smooth muscle cells of the arterial wall
4) cell death and injury
5) the formation of a necrotic, lipid-rich (cholesterol-rich) core

Although the exact cause-and-effect relationships are not yet clear, what is clear is that atherosclerosis and the accompanying higher incidences of heart and blood vessel diseases exist in persons with many of the known risk factors.

As we examine some of the known risk factors, keep in mind that atherosclerosis has been implicated as the primary cause of most heart and blood vessel diseases. This condition accounts for more than 800,000 heart attack and stroke deaths annually in the United States. This number is significant when one considers that for every death resulting from an accident, seven or eight persons die of stroke or heart attack.

Genetically controlled risk factors There are a few risk factors over which the individual has no control. These include family history (genetic susceptibility), the aging process and sex.

The *family history* of a person is an important risk factor, particularly when one or both parents had premature (before age 60) heart attacks. One should pay special attention to this risk factor if one's grandparents also had premature heart disease.

In rare instances one inherits a disorder known as hypercholesterolemia (a blood lipid metabolic disorder). This condition seriously increases one's risk and requires medical attention. In addition, such a disorder requires that the individual evaluate and control as many other risk factors as possible.

Although family traits predispose one to heart disease, the causal agents are not always clear. For example, children who smoke, have poor diets, are obese and are sedentary often have parents who exhibit these same lifestyle behaviors. The socio-cultural influences, therefore, cannot be discounted even where hereditary susceptibility to premature heart disease is readily apparent. Likewise the absence of a family history of heart disease does not guarantee immunity.

According to the American Heart Association[11] *aging* is another known risk factor. That is, the prevalence of heart disease increases with age for both men and women.

In his discussion of risk factors, Dr. Henry Blackburn[12] contends that the aging process alone does not seem to cause coronary artery disease. He points out that many elderly persons in the United States and other regions of the world live to advanced ages with no evidence of atherosclerosis or heart disease.

Perhaps what is most significant in this discussion is that nearly twenty-five percent of all heart attacks occur before the age of sixty-five. Nevertheless, continual arterial exposure to a variety of lifestyle risk factors would normally increase the chance of heart disease manifesting itself in old age.

Sex is another known risk factor in heart disease. As a student in one of our classes asked, is it because of too much or too little? Actually, neither. It depends on whether you are male or female. American males, particularly white males, have far higher rates of heart disease than American women. The disease strikes men at younger ages, but women catch up at about sixty-five years of age.

Exactly what mechanism offers protection for women is not clear. Whether it is hormonal (as some speculation suggests) or whether it is environmentally induced remains to be determined. Whatever the reasons, the fact remains that an appalling number of men suffer from and die of heart disease in their thirties, forties and fifties in the United States.

Ethnic origin is sometimes cited as another possible heart disease risk factor. In the United States the rates of heart disease deaths are highest for white males. Although black males have lower death rates from heart disease, they have higher incidences of hypertension, which contributes to coronary artery disease and strokes.

Worldwide demographic studies of ethnic migration tend to rule out this hereditary factor. Indications are that heart disease is more dependent upon behavioral patterns and lifestyle habits formed in childhood than upon ethnic origin. Many of the studies indicate that adoption of a Western style of living also brings about an increase in the risk of developing cardiovascular diseases.

Medically controllable risk factors The risk of heart disease increases among individuals who have high blood pressure, are diabetic or have high blood lipid (fat) levels. Fortunately, these conditions can often be managed with medical treatment and dietary changes.

Hypertension (high blood pressure) is a medical problem when the systolic/diastolic readings (taken at rest) approach 140/90. Medication and a sodium-restricted diet are usually prescribed as the pressure readings approach or exceed 160/90. Normal ranges for blood pressure fall beneath 140/90, with an average of 120/80 considered normal mid-range.

There are no outward symptoms of high blood pressure. It is often called the silent disease because symptoms of pain and/or inflammation associated with other disorders are not present. Although there is a tendency to inherit hypertension, the exact cause of it is unknown in the majority of cases. This is called *essential* hypertension. Of the millions in the United States with hypertension, some know the cause. This is called *secondary* hypertension and could be due to kidney or other known disease.

In addition to drug treatment, a sodium-restricted diet and regular exercise are also prescribed. Most nutritionists do not know the exact relationship between high-salt diets and hypertension. However, most agree that the American diet is already supersaturated with sodium and reducing intake is advisable. Exercise which is regular, moderate and aerobic has been found helpful in reducing blood pressure for some hypertensives.

Diabetes is another controllable predisposing condition. The fluctuating levels of blood sugar (glucose) and the often overweight condition of the diabetic seem to be the sources of trouble.

Most diabetics under medical supervision have been able to control their disorder and live relatively normal lives. Close monitoring of diets and the use of insulin will enable the diabetic to reduce and/or control this known risk factor.

Elevated blood *cholesterol* level is another modifiable risk factor for most individuals. Research implicating cholesterol in heart disease comes from the extensive study carried out among the population of Framingham, Massachusetts[13] and other studies. At the Aerobics Research Institute, Dr. Kenneth Cooper[14] considers a cholesterol level above 250 mg % a definite risk.

But there is more to the cholesterol story. It is known that the body manufactures cholesterol (in the liver) and that it is an essential component of body cells. Careful testing has also discovered that there are several different types of cholesterol and they are packaged differently for transport in the blood. Researchers generally have found that the Low Density Lipoprotein (LDL) variety is more apparent in heart diseased individuals than the High Density Lipoprotein (HDL) variety. Some serious exercise researchers have discovered high levels of HDL in young women and in individuals who engage in regular aerobic-type exercise.

The exact relationship between the development of atherosclerosis and cholesterol will become clear with additional research. This research may also reveal why increased levels of HDL offer a protective effect against atherosclerosis.

Medical treatment can assist in lowering the cholesterol level. But treatment often consists of dietary modification. This modification includes lowering the intake of cholesterol-rich foods such as eggs and reducing sugar intake.

Personally controlled risk factors The Secretary of Health and Human Services, Richard Schweiker, made front-page headlines in the Baltimore *Evening Sun* on October 30, 1982 where he was quoted as saying that "unhealthy lifestyles" are the leading cause of death in the United States.

In his address at a Johns Hopkins University conference, Schweiker noted that more federal funds will be devoted to promote exercise, healthier diets and instill the concept of wellness in the American people. He indicated that a health-conscious middle-aged American man can expect to live eleven years longer than his unhealthy, unfit colleague.

The personally controlled risk factors include inadequate diets (including obesity), smoking, stress and lack of appropriate exercise. The significant consideration about these factors is that they involve personal habits. Often these acquired behaviors are misinterpreted as innate or as natural developments, because it is usually next to impossible to change these old habits. But in a real sense these factors are not innate and an individual *does* have the capability to change or modify them.

Diets which are not nutritionally balanced, which contain more sodium (salt), sugar, triglycerides (saturated fats) and cholesterol than the body needs, or which have excess calories and thus cause obesity (too much fat) are contributing factors in heart and blood vessel diseases. According to Dr. Kenneth Cooper in *The Aerobics Way*,[15] thirty-six percent of the known risk factors are related to diet.

Since each person has direct control over what is put into the mouth, these conditions can be modified by changing one's eating patterns. This process certainly is not easy for everyone— old habits are indeed not easy to change. The change must begin by personally assessing how important these dietary changes are with respect to your health and your self-image. More about nutrition and weight control will be detailed in a later chapter.

Smoking is a factor which doubles the rate of heart disease for smokers as compared to non-smokers. Although many adults have quit smoking, the habit is still very popular among teenagers, especially young girls. Smoking is particularly harmful to individuals who have one or more other risk factors.

Smoking seems to have a role to play in the proliferation of atherosclerosis. The nicotine in cigarettes constricts arteries while the smoker's blood oxygen level is reduced. This occurs because the carbon monoxide in the smoke tends to have a greater affinity for red blood cells (hemoglobin) than oxygen.

It should be mentioned that this process takes place gradually and normally in individuals who have smoked for many years. Because the smoking habit is difficult to end, it is advisable not to start in the first place. Furthermore, lung cancer is the leading cause of cancer deaths in men and the second-leading cause of cancer deaths in women. The evidence linking heavy smoking to lung cancer is nearly irrefutable.

Lack of Exercise is another contributing risk factor. Sedentary individuals tend to carry more fat on their bodies than active individuals. Inactive people handle sudden excessive physical exertion less effectively than their fit counterparts. They fatigue more rapidly and have less energy to perform repetitive tasks. In addition they are more injury-prone because they lack the muscular strength, endurance and agility resulting from regular exercise. Cooper's research again demonstrates that individuals who do poorly on his exercise treadmill test are at a much higher risk than those who score well on the test.

Regular and moderate exercises which include an aerobic component are the most beneficial in reducing coronary disease risks. These are exercises of moderation by which the body gradually improves its ability to use large quantities of oxygen. Aerobic exercises have a direct and beneficial effect upon the heart and blood vessels.

Activities which appear to be most beneficial in this regard include walking, cycling, jogging, running, swimming and sports where the activity is continuous. Activities such as sprint running and weight lifting are anaerobic—that is, they are too intense and of too short a duration. Sports such as bowling and slow dancing are recreational, and therefore they have low aerobic value.

Since this is essentially a book on physical fitness, the various types of aerobic, anaerobic and non-aerobic activities are described in detail in other chapters.

Stress, the pressures we all face in our daily lives, is another controllable heart disease risk factor. Investigations by Drs. Friedman and Rosenman[16] led them to conclude that stress was the major cause of heart disease. They contend that the risk of heart disease doubles in persons with what they call Type A behaviors compared to the more easy-going persons identified as Type B.

Most authorities list stress as another important risk factor, but few agree that it is the primary factor. Most do agree that long-term, uncontrolled stress can lead to severe and debilitating disorders, including heart disease. A more detailed chapter discussing stress as a major health problem is included in this book.

ASSESSING YOUR RISK FACTORS

Now that you have reviewed some of the more important risk factors, it is essential that you assess your own risks. By identifying your potential risks, you can set realistic goals which will help you reduce them.

As you examine your heart disease risk profile, remember that many of the factors are behavioral and are directly under your control. That is not to suggest that these negative health behaviors are easily changed. They are not—changing habits is never easy. But if you are to begin a sound personal health program to reduce your chances of a chronic illness, you have little choice. With professional assistance when necessary, and a serious commitment to change, you can modify and control these health behaviors.

Several simple survey instruments are available to help you identify your risk factors. One popular one, known as the Arizona Heart Test,[17] was aired on the ABC television program *20/20* in February 1981. This program was of such interest to the American public that over 230,000 people returned their results to the Arizona Heart Institute. Other tests, such as Dr. Zohman's questionnaire,[18] the RISKO survey, and Cooper's Coronary Risk Profile, will help you compare results with the Arizona Test.

Give the test to yourself and discuss the results with your personal physician or other medical professional. Remember that these are not definitive tests of heart disease—only follow-up medical tests can verify the extent of your risks. If you are unsure about specific factors such as diabetes, your blood pressure, or your triglyceride and cholesterol levels, tests for these are often given at relatively low cost by public health or community health agencies.

The old adage about "an ounce of prevention" being worth "a pound of cure" has never been more important than it is today. Go for it!

REDUCING RISKS

If in the course of assessing your risk factors you have identified one or more which require attention, do not hesitate to take personal action. As indicated previously, your initial step is to consult with your physician. Your doctor can assist directly with helping you reduce or control specific medical problems.

Your doctor can also advise you about how to reduce or control factors which are non-medical or behavioral in nature. But remember, it is your responsibility to change your lifestyle, not your doctor's. If you cannot go it alone, seek out the programs or support groups which exist in every community and which will motivate you and commit you to a desirable change.

Perhaps Dr. Paul Dudley White's commitment to heart disease prevention will inspire you. He wrote:

> It was during the decade of the 1950s that I realized and preached by voice and by pen that the prevention of heart disease should have the first priority over diagnosis and treatment, vital though those were.[21]

Many of us have health responsibilities to others besides ourselves. For example, parents must take a more active role in participating and assisting children in preventive health measures. Poor diet and exercise habits often begin early in life.

Because children are subjected to the same lifestyles as their parents, researchers have begun to evaluate the risk factors in young children. In programs such as the Heart Watch Program, under the direction of Dr. Bill Tomek at Cortland State University in New York, many children have been observed to have one or more risk factors.

Studies conducted on American soldiers killed in Korea and Vietnam indicated that atherosclerosis was already present in many twenty-year-olds. These and other such studies are clear indications that the sedentary habits of children (such as too much passive television watching) and early diet programs could account for the high incidence of coronary artery disease in the United States.

Undoubtedly efforts to prevent risk must begin with very young children. For this to happen, of course, parents must become actively involved in the prevention process. One of the best ways is for parents to set an example.

POST-CORONARY EXERCISE

Survivors of heart attacks naturally worry about their future—their jobs, their families, their ability to live an active life. On the advice of their physicians and friends, many have joined exercise rehabilitation programs.

Others have avoided such programs because of the fear that physical exertion may precipitate a second heart attack or because it is not convenient for them. The main question for the post-coronary patient is: Will exercise be beneficial?

Most physicians who have participated in the development of such exercise programs throughout the United States would answer with an emphatic "yes." Most would also agree that exercise may be contraindicated for a small percentage of former heart attack victims. However, the results observed and follow-up studies over the past fifteen years suggest that patients benefit both physically and psychologically from these programs.

Moderate aerobic exercise and modification of other risk factors, such as diet and stress, help reduce the odds against a second attack and increase survivability if one does occur.

Hundreds of post-cardiac rehabilitation programs exist in the United States. Some are affiliated with hospitals. Many YMCA's sponsor programs. Others are privately administered. Perhaps the least expensive ones have been organized by local community colleges.

Catonsville Community College in Maryland organized a program called P.A.C.E. (Prescribed Active Cardiac Exercise) in 1974. The program was in cooperation with Union Memorial and St. Agnes Hospitals in Baltimore. Other area colleges followed with programs of their own. Most programs are directly supervised by highly trained exercise specialists and medical personnel.

The Toronto Rehabilitation Program In 1967 the Toronto Rehabilitation Centre, under the direction of Dr. Terence

Kavanaugh, was one of the first programs to emphasize endurance-type exercise. Dr. Kavanaugh's work became world famous because of the courageous effort of seven of his heart patients. On April 15, 1973, seven middle-aged Canadians from the "sickest track club in the world" finished the Boston Marathon. Herman Robers completed the event in four hours and thirty-two minutes.

Through gradual and progressive aerobic exercise training, these men were able to run twenty-six miles and 385 yards—an incredible feat even for healthy hearts.

Trained under the careful eye of Dr. Kavanaugh and monitored throughout the marathon run, this effort demonstrated that individuals can become fit despite heart disease. Dr. Kavanaugh explains his program in great detail in his book *Heart Attack: Counter-Attack.*[22]

Coronary exercise programs may not reverse the atherosclerotic development underlying coronary artery disease, but many patients participating in these programs have altered and now control many previously known risk factors and have greatly improved their functional capacities to exercise. Some make no gains in physical fitness but report a new zest for living because of the psychological benefits resulting from the regular participation and camaraderie which exist in most programs.

EXERCISE AND PREVENTION OF HEART DISEASE

Those who work in the Physical Development Center at Catonsville Community College always know when one of their colleagues had a heart attack. The sedentary administrative and faculty co-workers become visible as they frantically start their jogging programs—again! Following an enthusiastic effort for several days, and sometimes several weeks, the out-of-shapers again disappear, only to reappear following another heart attack announcement.

When asked why they stopped coming to the gym, the usual response was that they were just too busy and could not fit it into their schedules. The fear was gone once again—unfortunately, too many people start exercise programs because of a "fear" that if they don't they may have a heart attack. With fear as the prime motivator, the effort dissipates as rapidly as the fear subsides.

On the other hand, motivation to exercise may result from a sincere desire to reduce stress, improve one's figure, enhance one's self-image, improve a sports skill, or simply feel better. These programs often last.

Regardless of your motivation to exercise, a fair question to ask is: How effective is exercise in preventing a heart attack? Hard scientific evidence does not give all the answers to this complex question. However, presumptive evidence demonstrates clearly that regular and appropriate exercise is a prudent preventive measure. Moreover, there is significant evidence and staggering statistics to demonstrate the opposite effect.

Many cardiologists who also work extensively in the exercise field do answer the question of effectiveness. In 1979 Zohman, Kattus and Softness wrote:

> We have believed for many years that strenuous physical exercise is so beneficial that it helps to prevent heart attacks . . . but we don't exactly know yet how and why regular physical exercise helps prevent heart attacks.[23]

Dr. Kenneth Cooper puts it this way:

> I hope we do get the evidence, some day, that the right diet and exercise can be a *cure* for heart disease. But right now I want to make it clear that there is evidence that preventive medicine will work, in the overwhelming majority of cases, to *prevent* or delay the onset of heart disease—to help you *survive* a heart attack—and to help immeasurably to *rehabilitate* you following a heart attack.[24]

Medical research will continue to unravel the specific cause and effect relationships between exercise and degenerative diseases, particularly atherosclerosis-caused coronary heart disease. If you are inactive and have other risk factors, you cannot afford to wait for definitive answers. You must begin a program now based on the best available information.

EXERCISE AND LONGEVITY

We have all heard the story of the ninety-year-old person who remarked, "If I had known I was going to live this long I would have taken better care of myself." This sounds like a George Burns quotation. Actually, George did give a sound piece of advice about getting old on a recent television show when he stated that you can't help getting old, but you don't have to *get* old.

The secrets of living a long life are at best elusive. Even those who have survived into their nineties and hundreds give varying opinions of why they lived so long. However, there appears to be a common theme to their attitudes about long life.

Most of them have zest and an exuberance for a high-quality yet simplified existence, filled with love for the small mysteries and beauties of life. And often their determination includes an intense motivation to remain physically active and vibrant. They are participants in life, not spectators of it.

As our population of senior citizens grows and rightfully becomes more active publicly, we shall witness a continual increase in the average life span. Many of our crowded fitness programs for seniors also attest to their supreme interest in physical activity.

Although we may not have all of the "secrets" to longevity, we have sufficient evidence of premature deaths because of factors that don't work. We are now familiar with these risk factors, but what about exercise and longevity? Will exercise make a difference?

Individuals just beginning a program of exercise ask whether they will live longer if they exercise, implying that if the answer is "yes" then they will really work hard. If the answer is "no" or "maybe," they will perhaps have a good excuse when they discontinue the program. After all, if exercise is not going to enable a person to live longer, then why spend all that effort and sweat in such a futile struggle?

Unfortunately for those who start exercising *because* it will make them live longer, science has no definitive answers. The opinion of some experts should nonetheless be taken seriously.

McArdle, Katch and Katch state:

> Because older fit individuals have many of the functional characteristics of younger people, one could argue that improved physical fitness may help retard the aging process and thus offer some protection to health in later life.[15]

The September 1979 issue of *The Physician and Sports Medicine* reported a full-length discussion of the relationship of exercise to cardiovascular disease and longevity. Dr. Shepard's closing statement sums up the longevity question and offers a good piece of advice for all of us:

> Adding up the primary and secondary mechanisms, I think the evidence suggests quite strongly that exercise is going to extend life. For those who want to take the gamble, it is a good one.[16]

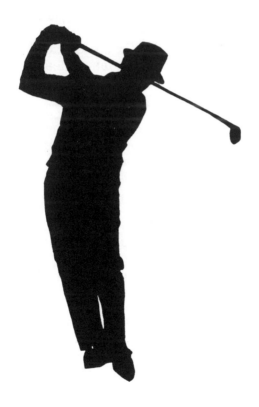

The evidence suggests that exercise is going to extend life.

REFERENCES

1. Sheehan, George, *Dr. Sheehan on Running*. Mountain View, CA.: World Publications, 1975, p. 85.
2. Davis, Goode P., Edward Park and Editors of U.S. News Books, *The Heart: The Living Pump*. Washington, D.C., 1981.
3. Fisher, Arthur, and the editors of Time-Life Books, *The Healthy Heart*. Alexandria, VA.: Time-Life Books, 1981.
4. White, Paul Dudley, *My Life and Medicine*. Boston: Gambitt Publishers, 1971.
5. Cooper, Kenneth, *Aerobics*. New York: M. Evans and Company, 1968. (Also a Bantam paperback.)
6. *The Journal of Physical Education,* "Special Report: Proceedings of the National YMCA Consultation on Cardiovascular Health," Summer 1976, p. 137.
7. Debakey, Michael and Antonio Gotto, *The Living Heart*. New York: Charter Books, 1977, p. 157.
8. American Heart Association, *Heart Facts*. Dallas, American Heart Association, 1983.
9. American Heart Association, *Heartbook*. New York: Dutton, 1980, p. 17.
10. Cooper, Kenneth, *The Aerobics Way*. New York: M. Evans and Company, 1977 (and Bantam Books).
11. Friedman, Meyer, and Ray H. Rosenman, *Type A Behavior and Your Heart*. New York: Fawcett-Crest Books, 1974.
12. Dietrich, Edward B., *The Arizona Heart Institute's Heart Test*. New York: Cornerstone Library (Simon and Schuster), 1981.
13. Zohman, Lenore R., Albert A. Kattus and Donald G. Softness, *The Cardiologist's Guide to Fitness and Health Through Exercise*. New York: Simon and Schuster, 1979, pp. 36-37.
14. Kavanaugh, Terence, *Heart Attack? Counter-Attack!* Toronto: Van Nostrand Reinhold, Ltd., 1976.
15. McArdle, William D., Frank I. Katch and Victor L. Katch, *Exercise Physiology: Energy, Nutrition, and Human Performance*. Philadelphia: Lea & Febiger, 1981, p. 430.
16. *The Physician and Sportsmedicine*, Vol. 7, No. 9, September, 1979, pp. 56-71.

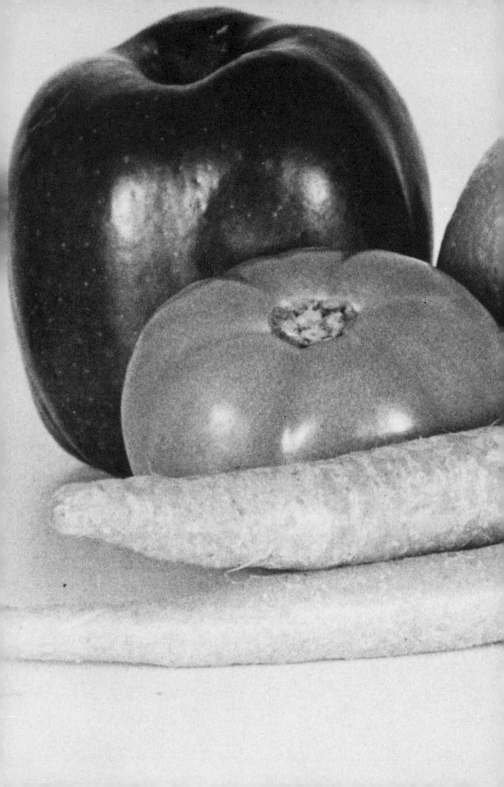

7

NUTRITION AND FITNESS

> I am not slender by nature, but by
> design and constant vigilance.
> > Nutrition expert
> > Jane Brody

OBJECTIVES

- List the six basic nutrient groups and describe the contribution each one makes toward good nutrition.

- Describe the process of digestion and how food is converted into useful energy by the body.

- Describe the importance of balancing nutrients and calories when designing a daily diet program.

- Examine the reasons why excessive salt, sugar, cholesterol and saturated fat intake may contribute to poor nutrition.

- Examine the typical daily diets of midshipmen and discuss how their diets relate to their overall fitness program.

- Identify and discuss several of the more common ideas regarding diet and nutrition for athletes.

Most of us have access to more nutritionally balanced and tasteful diets than any other nation on earth. Yet Americans in general have poor nutrition and dietary habits.

Our food selection is influenced mainly by television advertisements and our family traditions, rather than what is best for good health. We eat too much of non-nutrient foods such as sugar (over 100 pounds per year are consumed per person in the U.S.), which simply adds calories to our diets. We pump our bodies full of more salt than is necessary for good health. Our stores are lined with attractively packaged manufactured foods, most of which have questionable nutrient value.

In contrast to our overeating habits, we are also the most diet-conscious nation on earth. To the impartial observer our behavior appears ludicrous. We spend nearly twenty percent of our average family budget on food, then spend more money on diet programs to lose the fat we gained from overeating.

A word to the wise is usually sufficient, but not in the U.S.—if we practiced good eating habits and weight control habits, we would not have to spend billions of dollars a year to learn how to lose weight. Diet books are best-sellers in our bookstores and book clubs, and diet industries have literally exploded in the American business circles. Each new book or program promises us the magical way to lose excess pounds and keep them off.

If we eventually were to come to our sense about diet, we would realize that we can eat for pleasure—or for a host of other conscious or subconscious reasons—and still eat our way to good health. The foundation of a good nutrition program,however, is a basic knowledge about foods and how they are utilized by the body.

ESSENTIAL NUTRIENTS

Our bodies require six basic nutrients for good health. These include the three major food sources—carbohydrates, fats and proteins. In addition, our bodies require three other nutrients which enable us to effectively use the three major food sources—these include vitamins, minerals and water.

All six nutrients must be supplied to the body in the right proportions and correct amounts to achieve optimal nutritional health. Although nutrition is a relatively young science and confusion often results when different viewpoints are expressed, nutritionists in general are in agreement regarding the balance of nutrients. Let us define each nutrient and briefly examine its importance in the nutrient balance framework.

Carbohydrates By dissecting the word carbohydrate, one readily determines that it has something to do with carbon and water (hydrate). In fact, carbohydrates consist of the three elements carbon, hydrogen and oxygen—and most of us know that H_2O is the chemical symbol for water.

Most of the carbohydrate foods we consume come from plants or from products originating from plants. These would include all fresh vegetables and fruits, and also include bread, spaghetti and sugar, which are by-products derived from plants. We sometimes refer to carbohydrates as sugars or starches. A starch such as a potato is simply a food source made up of many molecules of simple sugars. Some carbohydrates (mainly simple sugars) are contained in the non-plant foods we eat. Honey and milk sugar are examples of non-plant carbohydrates.

When we eat carbohydrates, various digestive enzymes reduce them to their simplest component for their absorption into the bloodstream. In the blood these broken-down sugars and starches are known as glucose or blood sugar. All cells of the body (especially muscle cells) readily accept glucose and use it as the primary source of energy to perform cellular work.

By overeating (taking in more calories than we need) we greatly increase the blood glucose level. Since the body prefers not to waste this source of energy, it forms pods of sugar molecules called glycogen (body starch) and stores it in the muscles and the liver. When necessary, the body may call upon these reserve stores of energy by converting the glycogen back into usable glucose molecules.

If the stores of glucose and glycogen are full, the body also has the capacity to convert glucose into fat and store it in the fat "warehouses," such as those under the skin. Again, these fat stores represent a high grade of energy for the body whenever the need arises.

Fats Foods containing fats are derived from plant as well as animal products. Interestingly, fats contain the same three chemical elements as carbohydrates, namely carbon, hydrogen and oxygen. The chemical structure, of carbohydrates and fats are vastly different, however. A simple carbohydrate sugar may contain only six carbon atoms, whereas a simple fat may contain a chain of 36 carbon atoms with the hydrogen and oxygen atoms arranged quite differently. Largely because of the more complex arrangements of fat molecules, it is important to remember that fat also contains about twice as many calories (units of energy) as carbohydrate.

Animal meats and animal by-products, such as milk, contain fats known as saturated fats. Plants, on the other hand, contain fats known as unsaturated or poly-unsaturated fats. "Unsaturated" essentially means that the chemical bonds are not fully saturated with hydrogen. In practical terms, fats which are solid at room temperature, such as butter or leftover bacon grease, are saturated fats. Unsaturated fats usually remain in liquid form at room temperature. The controversy regarding the use of saturated versus unsaturated fats in one's diet will be discussed in the next chapter.

Most nutritionists do not recommend that fats be eliminated from your diet, as some weight loss programs suggest. Fats are an important source of energy for your body and also provide four essential vitamins, namely A, D, E and K. The fat-like substance cholesterol is also essential to the body but normally can be reduced in the diet because the body manufactures cholesterol on its own. More about cholesterol later.

Proteins The third major food source is protein. Once again, proteins contain the same three elements (carbon, hydrogen and oxygen) that are present in carbohydrates and fats. Unlike fats and carbohydrates, however, proteins also contain a fourth element—nitrogen.

Because carbohydrates, fats and proteins contain the same chemical elements (although in different configurations), all three are possible sources of cellular energy. Protein is not used as readily as fats and carbohydrates for normal energy needs. Remember, however, that if we consume an abundance of any of the three, the excess can easily be converted into fat and stored in our bodies.

The nitrogen component of protein gives it a unique quality that fats and carbohydrates do not have—it allows protein to be used in the growth and repair of human tissue. Nitrogen is contained in protein's simpler molecules, called amino acids, which are essential and vital to all of life's processes. over twenty have been identified, and eight must be obtained directly from the foods we eat. The remaining amino acids are manufactured by the body. It is easy to understand the extreme significance of proteins if we consider that DNA and RNA, the substances which carry our genetic codes, are formed by amino acids derived from proteins.

Foods containing proteins include those from animal origins like meat, poultry and fish. Proteins also occur in plant sources such as cereals and vegetables. One should eat a variety of foods to assure adequate supply of all amino acids.

Vitamins These are very small organic compounds which are essential to the normal functioning of the body's metabolic processes. They act as catalysts for the biochemical events occurring in the body, and the absence of specific vitamins can cause serious illness and even death. Taking too many vitamins can also be hazardous to your health.

Vitamins are generally categorized as either water-soluble or fat-soluble. The fat-soluble vitamins are A, D, E and K. All other vitamins are water-soluble. The table on page 196 identifies the known vitamins and their specific functions. Vitamins are obtained from a broad spectrum of foods, and therefore any diet should include a large variety of foods.

Vitamins can also be obtained in manufactured (synthetic) forms. Some controversy exists about whether it is more healthful to take vitamins in the synthetic form or in the food we eat. The "natural" argument focuses on the point that vitamins are more useful to the body when taken in combinations with other natural nutrients contained in the food we eat.

It is important to remember that vitamins are essential to good health when they are taken in the right amounts. Vitamin deficiency can cause serious illnesses. On the other hand, the over-ingestion of certain vitamins can also be toxic to the body. The attitude that because a little is good, more must be better simply is not true with vitamins or any other nutrient. The use of mega-vitamin doses for the healthy person or the serious athlete is currently considered imprudent. There are occasions when vitamin mega-doses are recommended for a certain disorder, but these should always be prescribed by a physician.

Minerals Minerals are inorganic substances required by the body in very small amounts. They aid metabolic processes and are important building materials of body tissue. Some are metallic substances such as iron and copper. Others, such as iodine and sodium, are non-metallic.

Functions and Sources of Essential Nutrients

Nutrient	Function	Problems associated with deficiency	Source
Calories	Supply energy for growth and development and normal body functioning.	Inadequate caloric intake in children is evidenced by lack of growth and energy and loss of weight.	All foods. Starchy, sweet, and fat foods are concentrated sources.
Protein	Essential for normal growth and development.	A severe or prolonged deficiency in children results in retarded growth and may retard mental development. In adults, deficiency symptoms (weight loss, lassitude, and decreased resistance to disease) are less specific.	Foods of animal origin, namely, meat, fish, poultry and milk products. Cereals and beans are also an important source of protein.
Vitamin A	Essential for the formation of cells, particularly in the skin, and for normal vision; aids in maintaining resistance to infections.	Deficiency signs: Night blindness, and skin changes characterized by dry, rough skin. Prolonged vitamin A deficiency can lead to permanent blindness.	Whole milk and whole-milk products; dark-green, leafy, and yellow vegetables; liver.
Vitamin D	Necessary for the absorption of calcium and the normal development of bones.	Lack of vitamin D causes rickets in children.	Vitamin D—fortified milk. Vitamin D is formed in the skin upon exposure to sunlight.
Vitamin C	Important for normal tooth and bone formation and wound healing. Plays a role in normal resistance to infection.	Deficiency results in soft, spongy gums, prolonged wound healing, and in the advanced deficiency state, the classical disease scurvy.	Citrus fruits, tomatoes, and certain vegetables such as cabbage and potatoes.
Thiamin	Essential for growth, normal function of the nervous system, and normal metabolism.	Deficiency results in retarded growth, edema, and changes in the nervous system. Advanced deficiency can result in beriberi.	Liver, eggs, whole grain or enriched cereals and cereal products, and lean meat.

Functions and Sources of Essential Nutrients, Cont.

Nutrient	Function	Problems associated with deficiency	Source
Riboflavin	Essential for utilization of protein and is also involved in other metabolic processes.	Deficiency can result in skin changes such as angular lesions, tongue changes, and poor growth.	Dairy products are the major source, but meats and green leafy vegetables are other sources.
Niacin	Essential for normal digestion and utilization of food.	The classical deficiency state is pellagra, characterized by diarrhea, dermatitis, dementia, and death.	Liver, meats, whole grain, and enriched cereals and cereal products.
Calcium	Necessary for formation of bones and teeth. Also plays a role in normal blood clotting and normal functioning of nerve tissue.	Deficiency in children may be associated with rickets; in adults, calcium may be lost from the bones.	Milk and milk products, fortified cereal products, and certain leafy vegetables.
Iron	Necessary for the formation of hemoglobin, a component of red blood cells.	Iron deficiency symptoms include weakness and fatigability. Advanced deficiency leads to anemia.	Liver, green leafy vegetables, dried fruits, enriched cereals and cereal products, molasses, and raisins.
Iodine	Essential for normal function of the thyroid gland.	Deficiency results in an enlargement of the thyroid gland, which is known as goiter.	Iodized salt is probably the most widely used source. Seafood, water, and plants from certain areas contribute substantial amounts.

Source: *Ten-State Nutrition Survey 1967-70*, vol. 1, U.S. Department of Health, Education, and Welfare, p. 4.

Human life as we know it could not exist without the presence of minerals such as sodium, calcium, chlorine, iron, magnesium, phosphorous and potassium. Neither could life exist without traces of the micro-minerals such as cobalt, chromium, copper, iodine, selenium and others.

Diets which lack a variety of foods may not provide the small amounts of minerals required by the body. In fact, the diet may in some instances appear to be balanced and to contain all minerals, but for some reason the body is not accepting the mineral. The only way to check this is to have a periodic blood analysis to determine the actual levels present. Your physician therefore can be a great help to you if you are mineral deficient and require mineral supplementation.

Water It is not possible to survive more than several days without water, an essential nutrient which must be consumed regularly throughout each day to replace the water lost through the skin, urine and respiration.

Every metabolic process occurring in the body requires the presence of water. As these processes speed up, such as during vigorous exercise, water intake must be increased to offset the increased loss through sweating. Dehydration, especially for distance runners, is a common concern but can be avoided with proper safeguards.

As an essential nutrient, water must be considered an important factor in good nutrition. When we discuss physical fitness and exercise throughout the book, the specific role of water will be examined. For the weight-conscious person it should be remembered that water contains zero calories.

CONVERTING FOOD INTO USEFUL ENERGY

Persons interested in fitness should have at least a superficial understanding of how the food we eat directly affects bodily functions both at rest and during exercise. A better understanding of the process should help to alleviate some of the misunderstandings and myths regarding nutrition and physical performance.

A simplistic analysis of the process whereby the food we eat is converted into useful energy is as follows: 1) digestion, or the initial breakdown of food into smaller chemical units; 2) absorption of these smaller units into the bloodstream; 3) transportation of the food nutrients directly to the cells or to intermediate "factories" for further breakdown; 4) absorption of the molecules into cells and the subsequent release of energy to perform cellular work; and 5) discharge of waste products from the cells and eventually from the body. Several of these processes will be described briefly.

Individuals interested in a more detailed study of the biochemical processes of energy during human performance are referred to the recent exercise physiology text written by McKardle, Katch and Katch.

Digestion The first stage of changing the food we eat into sources of energy is called digestion. Throughout our digestive system (particularly the mouth, stomach and small intestines) substances called enzymes break food substances into smaller chemical units. In addition to these enzymes, powerful hydrochloric acid in the stomach and specific pancreatic and liver secretions also assist the digestive process. The esophagus and the colon (large intestines) are mainly passageways for food but have other minor functions as well.

Transport After food sources are digested into simpler molecules such as amino acids, simple sugars and fatty acids, they are absorbed into the bloodstream. This occurs mainly in the small intestines. Some substances, such as alcohol, are absorbed through the stomach wall, however.

These substances are then transported by the blood to tissues throughout the body. The liver is important during this phase of metabolism. It is here that intermediate metabolism of partially broken down fats occurs, mainly through the secretion of bile. The liver, the largest organ in the body also plays an important role in carbohydrate, protein, and vitamin production as well as in other life-sustaining functions.

Transport of energy sources to the cellular level is primarily through the blood. The cells then use this energy to perform specialized physiological work, such as causing muscles to contract, nerve tissue to transmit impulses, glands to secrete, tissue to grow and repair itself and the heart and brain to function with very little rest.

Because our interest in this book is primarily physical fitness, our focus will be upon how muscle cells oxidize carbohydrates and fats as the primary energy sources. Protein is very important in the growth and repair of muscle tissue, but it is not a significant contributor to the cell as an energy source.

Cellular metabolism Knowing how energy is released at the cellular level is important to the person interested in improving physical fitness. First, significant benefits from an exercise program are achieved when one understands how foods provide energy for muscular exertion. Secondly, knowing how metabolic pathways are activated in muscle cells influences the selection of training methods for the different types of fitness desired. Furthermore, understanding cellular metabolism is particularly important to the person who wishes to control weight.

The body is unable to stockpile large quantities of carbohydrates. Aside from what is present as blood glucose, Sharkey[2] estimates that the liver can store approximately 80 grams, and 15 grams are stored in each kilogram (2.2 pounds) of skeletal muscle. In the average male this amounts to about 1,200 calories of carbohydrate energy, which could fuel a ten-mile run. Because brain and nerve metabolism use only glucose for fuel, it is apparent that the body must carefully conserve its limited supplies of carbohydrates. Also remember that to replenish the supply used up, our daily intake of carbohydrates should exceed 50 percent of all calories eaten daily.

Fat, on the other hand, is the body's most abundant source of energy. The body's capacity to store fat is seemingly unlimited. Fat is the body's high octane fuel—it contains twice as much energy (calories) as an equal quantity of carbohydrate. Sharkey estimates that a person with 30 pounds of fat (eg. a 120-pound female with 24% body fat) would have enough fuel to run more than 1,000 miles.[3]

The roles which carbohydrates (glucose and glycogen) and fats (fatty acids) play as energy sources during various intensities of exercise become clearer when the concept of aerobic and anaerobic cellular metabolism is understood. "Anaerobic" means without oxygen and "aerobic" means with oxygen.

Muscular work can be powered by cellular substances without the presence of oxygen. Such intense anaerobic work can only last for a short time because the immediate energy sources (namely ATP and glycogen) cannot be reconstituted quickly enough to maintain muscular effort. On the other hand, during aerobic work a sufficient supply of oxygen is present in this complex metabolic system to reconstitute large amounts of ATP. ATP (adenosintriphosphate) is essential for muscular work, and the energy delivered from the oxidation of carbohydrates and fats is used to reconstitute ATP.

TIME

| 0s | 4s | 10s | 1½ min | 3 min + |

ATP

Strength-power
power lift, high jump
shot put, golf swing, tennis serve

ATP-CP

**Sustained
power**
sprints, fast breaks, football line play

ATP-CP + Lactic Acid

**Anaerobic
Power-Endurance**
200-400m dash,
100-yard swim

Aerobic endurance
beyond ½ mile run

TYPES OF PERFORMANCE

Immediate/Short-Term
Non-Oxidative Systems

Aerobic-Oxidative
System

Predominant Energy Pathways

**Classification of activities based on duration of performance and the
predominant intracellular energy pathways.**

When aerobic work is compared to anaerobic work the ratio of ATP production is 38 to 2. In practical terms this means that aerobic work can go on indefinitely, whereas in anaerobic exertion (such as running an all-out sprint), fatigue sets in very rapidly. It is clear from this example that the body, therefore, uses more of its major source of energy (fat) to power aerobic exercise and reserves much of its limited energy source (glycogen) for anaerobic exercise.

Again, in practical terms, when one desires to improve aerobic fitness, the body must be trained to utilize larger quantities of oxygen and use larger quantities of fatty acids. Sprinters, on the other hand, must train their muscles to perform anaerobic work more efficiently. The Table on page 201 illustrates the types of metabolic pathways utilized during various types of physical exertion. The terms aerobic and anaerobic will be used again in the description of cardiovascular and muscular fitness.

A BALANCED DIET

How does one seeking a nutritious and healthful diet survive the information explosion? How are the facts separated from the myths, and how is the truth synthesized from the food advertising blitz we face daily on our television sets? Even the experts often disagree about what is and what is not good for us to eat.

Aside from the apparent controversy surrounding substances such as cholesterol, salt, sugar, saturated fats and food additives, there are some reasonable guidelines for us to follow. These guidelines include: 1) nutrient balancing, and 2) caloric balancing.

Nutrient balancing Nutritionists are in general agreement that the six basic nutrients described previously are essential to good health. Most would also agree that all the known nutrients must be in balance with all other nutrients. For this reason the U.S.A. Food and Nutrition Board (National Academy of Sciences National Research Council) has established RDA's (Recommended Daily Allowances) for persons of all ages in the United States. In addition, the U.S. Department of Agriculture has published excellent tables which list the nutrient values of nearly all types of food eaten in the United States.

While it would be very difficult for the average person to monitor and calculate the exact amounts of nutrients in an average diet, it is certainly possible to eat a varied diet. By avoiding a monotonous diet which is also nutrient-poor, and eating a variety of foods (generally following the four food-group guidelines), nutrient balancing is possible. For those who wish to be precise in their estimates, there are computer programs available that will do the laborious calculations.

Caloric balancing

For the nutrition-conscious person, caloric balance has several meanings.

First, it is recommended that calories obtained from carbohydrates, fats and proteins be balanced according to a ratio of the total number of calories consumed in an average day. For the non-dieter, the ratio of 50% carbohydrates, 30% fats and 20% proteins represents a good guideline, according to Cooper.[4] Others might scale the carbohydrates upward to 60-65% and the fats and proteins down by 5-10%. Most nutritionists would recommend that most of the carbohydrates consist of the complex starches and that the fats consist mostly of unsaturated varieties.

The second meaning of caloric balancing refers to maintenance of proper and stable body weight. Once one has achieved an "ideal" weight, the daily caloric intake should nearly equal the expenditure of calories if the weight is to remain stable. If one becomes more physically active, an upward adjustment of intake is required. On the other hand, if one becomes less physically active there should be a downward adjustment in caloric intake. In relatively simple terms, an imbalance of intake and output of calories leads to either a weight gain or a weight loss. Unfortunately most people in America become less active as they get older but forget to also lower their caloric intake proportionately.

Nutrition guidelines The U.S. Department of Agriculture dietary guidelines for Americans reflect a simple yet common-sense approach which reflects most of the recent nutrition research.[5] The guidelines were written for Americans who are already healthy. The special needs of infants, children with certain deficiencies, pregnant females, the aged and persons with other disorders or metabolic problems may need to vary these guidelines according to a physician-prescribed program. In general, competitive athletes can also effectively use the guidelines with perhaps a slight modification of total caloric intake to meet the demands of their particular sport. The guidelines are as follows:

1) Eat a variety of foods
2) Maintain ideal weight
3) Avoid too much fat, saturated fat and cholesterol
4) Eat foods with adequate starch and fiber
5) Avoid too much sugar
6) Avoid too much sodium
7) If you drink alcohol, do so in moderation

These general nutrition guidelines can be easily integrated into your daily routine. Eating will remain pleasurable and nutritionally sound without requiring inordinate amounts of time being spent in food preparation, calorie counting and nutrient balancing.

We must remember, however, that nutrition is a complex subject and does not have a long history of scientific investigation, and areas of controversy exist within the scientific and medical communities. As knowledge about nutrition grows through scientific pursuits, we can expect to see changes in most nutritional guidelines.

SPECIAL NUTRITION CONCERNS

Those areas of nutrition that are most confusing to the general public will be identified and briefly described.

Vitamins

Perhaps more confusion exists about vitamins than any other essential nutrient. The confusion is further compounded when widely publicized claims (usually from someone respected in the scientific community or a celebrity) links a vitamin with a miraculous improvement of health. Often, without medical consultation to determine whether a deficiency exists or a vitamin increase is warranted, millions of people seek the "magical cure" on their own.

Fortunately for most people who behave in this manner, the use of vitamin mega-doses to prevent colds, heart attacks or gout has no detrimental effect except on the pocketbook. Despite the vitamin's having no direct relationship to bodily changes, any improvement in feelings and attitude is enough to convince one that the vitamin indeed made the difference. The unfortunate fact is that mega-doses of certain vitamins are toxic and dangerous to the body.

This is not to say that vitamins are not directly or indirectly linked to specific disorders. Several hundred years ago the British Navy inadvertently discovered a connection between ascorbic vitamin C deficiency and the condition known as scurvy. Vitamin D is inextricably connected to the metabolism of calcium and phosphorus, and its deficiency causes rickets. However, moderation in dosage seems to be the general recommendation, and a varied diet is the best way to assure proper amounts of these important substances. Some physicians do recommend a one-a-day supplement because of the irregular eating patterns of many Americans.

Cholesterol The importance of cholesterol to good health has been known for some time. This fat-like (technically it is an alcohol, not a fat) substance is present in every human cell. Its function is to form the "skeletal" framework of each cell, including red blood cells. Without cholesterol each of us literally would become a "pile of protoplasmic mush."

Most research has demonstrated a relationship between high cholesterol levels and incidences of atherosclerosis. High cholesterol levels therefore are considered an important risk factor in heart and blood vessel disorders. The long-term Framingham study implicates cholesterol, although most researchers admit that the exact mechanism by which cholesterol and atherosclerosis are interconnected is not clear.

Recent scientific efforts are focusing on several types of cholesterol compounds. Actually cholesterol remains the same but is "trucked" differently throughout the body by substances known as lipoproteins. Four types of lipoproteins have been separated in the laboratory, but only two of them are of any significance to the cholesterol-atherosclerosis issue. They are high-density lipoprotein (HDL) and low-density lipoprotein (LDL).

In simplistic terms HDL is the "good" type of cholesterol and LDL the "bad" type. Studies indicate that young women and men of any age who engage in regular aerobic types of exercise have higher levels of HDL than do older women or men who do not exercise. In assessing cholesterol as a risk factor in heart disease, Cooper's findings indicate that the ratio of HDL to the *total* blood cholesterol is more important than the actual levels of HDL or LDL.[6]

As a normal, healthy adult, what advice would be appropriate to follow? Eat cholesterol in moderation and engage in a moderate aerobic exercise program to keep the HDL level up and the LDL level down. For children, unless they are predisposed to a condition known as hyperlipidemia or hypercholesterolemia, moderate intake of cholesterol is not considered harmful.

Saturated and unsaturated fats Dusek[7] recommends that the fat in our diets should not exceed 30 percent of the total caloric intake. She also recommends that for each gram of saturated fat in our diet two grams of unsaturated fat should be consumed.

Saturated fats are controversial because of their relationship to heart disease. As substances known as triglycerides, these fats are obtained largely from red meats. On the other hand, some polyunsaturated fats taken in large quantities seem to play a role in developing certain cancers. Although all answers are not yet clear, most nutritionists would recommend reducing the total fat consumed by Americans (estimated to be as high as 50%). But some intake of saturated and unsaturated fats is still essential for good health. Different fats have special roles to play in the metabolic and structural processes within the body. Oleic and linoleic unsaturated fats, for example, are essential in the diet because the body cannot synthesize them. Other dietary fats are essential because they contain the fat-soluble vitamins A, D, E and K.

Salt American diets contain too much salt, that is, more than what is needed for normal functioning of the body. Because salt is an important food preservative and taste enhancer, few processed or canned foods we eat are salt-free (sodium-free).

The sodium (salt) controversy exists principally because of the relationship between high salt levels and hypertensive disease (high blood pressure). As a major risk factor in heart disease and stroke, high blood pressure can also cause damage in other body organs such as the kidneys and eyes.

Again, what advice does the normally healthy person follow? Should everyone strive to have a sodium-restricted diet, or just those individuals with disorders requiring a restricted intake? The answer again perhaps lies in the word "moderation."

Salt deficiency from inadequate intake is extremely rare. Therefore, even by consciously avoiding high-sodium foods, you will recieve an adequate amount of sodium if your diet is balanced and includes a variety of foods. Recent research has also questioned whether athletes or those working in hot environments should take salt tablets. For these individuals, or for anyone who perspires freely, the most essential nutrient is water. Ample supplies of it should be taken to replace what is lost through perspiration and respiration.

Sugar Another subject of nutrition controversy is table sugar. Known as sucrose, this substance is the refined product made from sugar cane or sugar beets. Americans are weaned on sugar. We love its taste, and it is inexpensive to add to many foods processed for our consumption. We like it so much that an estimated one hundred-plus pounds of it are eaten every year by each person in the U.S. So why is sugar controversial?

First, table sugar contains calories (it is a simple carbohydrate), but no vitamins or minerals. Because it is a nutrient-empty food, we must get our nutrients entirely from other food sources. In the typical American diet this increases our caloric intake level—which leads to "creeping obesity."

A high intake of table sugar—such as we get from drinking a soda (some non-diet drinks contain up to eight teaspoons of sugar)—causes wild fluctuations in blood glucose. These give us abrupt mood and energy swings and may contribute to diabetes, hypoglycemia and possibly high triglyceride levels.

The opposing argument, which advocates taking in sugar from its natural food sources such as fruits, suggests that these sugars are digested and processed more slowly and efficiently by the body. The bonus is that you are able to obtain other important nutrients and fiber along with these natural sugars. These advocates would also argue that simple sugar is more likely to cause tooth decay than sugar contained in the more natural state.

In general, Americans would be practicing better nutrition habits by lowering their intake of table sugar products. What should you eat instead? Foods containing complex carbohydrates are healthy and should constitute about 80% of your carbohydrate intake.

Fiber Unlike cholesterol, salt and sugar, the concern is that there is too little fiber in the American diet. The trend toward eating more fast or processed foods has reduced our intake of natural food fiber, or roughage, as it was once called.

Fiber refers to the indigestible components of food. Fresh

fruits, vegetables and whole grains contain fibrous substances known as cellulose. Some writers refer to fiber as dietary bulk.

Adequate dietary fiber causes food to pass through the digestive system rapidly. Because fiber also absorbs water in the lower digestive track, there is less chance that various substances will irritate the colon. It is believed that diet and the food which passes through the digestive system are the direct cause of disorders of the bowel—intestinal and colon cancers, for example.

Because of the recent public discussion regarding the low fiber content in the American diet, food manufacturers are adding cellulose to juices, breads and pastries. Ordinarily a person will have ample fiber in the diet when a variety of fresh fruits, vegetables and whole grains (such as bran) are eaten regularly.

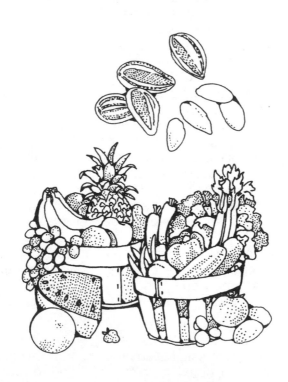

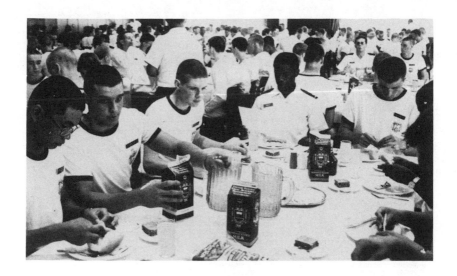

THE MIDSHIPMAN DIET

When do they eat? Meals at the U.S. Naval Academy are served to the midshipmen at regular intervals each day. Breakfast begins at 6:45 A.M., the noon meal at 12:20 P.M. and the evening meal at 6:30 P.M. Breakfast is required for all fourth classmen and optional for third, second and first classmen.

Where do they eat? All midshipmen assemble at mealtimes in the large King dining hall adjacent to their sleeping quarters. Food is prepared in the vast galley area and is served family style.

What do they eat? Careful analysis of the sample weekly menu for the midshipmen indicates that highly nutritious meals are served. There is careful balancing of carbohydrates, fats and proteins throughout the day and from day to day. The variety of food served throughout the week also assures that all essential proteins, vitamins and minerals are included in the diet. The menu also indicates the caloric value of the menu items to help the midshipmen generally regulate the total number of calories consumed.

Although midshipmen individually select their own food items from the menu, they are encouraged to eat a balanced selection of the items. This selection process assures adequate and necessary nutritional health to meet the rigors of daily life at the Academy.

UNITED STATES NAVAL ACADEMY
KING HALL

MENU FOR WEEK ENDING 13 February 1983

BREAKFAST	LUNCH	DINNER
"A" Watch - Mr. Duvall	**Monday 7 Feb. - Mr. Duvall**	**"B" Watch - Mr. Tubaya**
Orange Juice 8oz. 120C	Navy Bean Soup 1c. 175C	Weinersnitzel AvSv 600C
Assorted Cereal	Saltine Crackers	Tomato Gravy
Hot Hominy Grits ½c. 120C	Meatball Hero 600C	Scalloped Cheese Potatoes ½c. 250C
Fresh Apples	Hard Rolls	Fried Cabbage AvSv 60C
Scrambled Eggs ½c. 100C	Tater Wedges ¼c. 230C	Health Salad ½c. 150C
Broiled Bacon 1sl. 45C	Hearts of Lettuce	White Bread Butter
Plain Toast Butter	Ranch House/Caesar's Dressing	Carrot Cake W/Icing
Bran Muffins	Chocolate Chip Cookies ea. 100C	Hot Tea/Lemon Wedges
Hot Chocolate Coffee Milk	Grapeade Milk	Milk
"A" Watch - Mr. Duvall	**Tuesday 8 Feb. - Mr. Duvall**	**"B" Watch - Mr. Tubaya**
Grapefruit Juice 8oz. 90C	Mexican Meal W/ 325C	King Hall Fried Chicken 1 serv 500C
Assorted Cereal	Meat Filling	Chicken Gravy
Hot Oatmeal 1c. 130C	Taco Shells Taco Sauce	Mashed Potatoes ½c. 100C
Fresh Oranges	Shredded Lettuce/Cheese	Carrot Coins ½c. 40C
Breakfast Sandwich Kit W/ 420C	Chopped Tomatoes/Onions	Hearts of Lettuce 10C
Egg Omelet, Canadian Bacon,	Burritos 279C	Thousand Island/Caesar's Dressing
Sliced American Cheese, English Muffins	Nacho Cheese Sauce Doritos	White Bread Butter
Swedish Coffee Cake	Assorted Cup Cakes 235C	Paul Morisette Pie 1/6 cut 400C
Hot Chocolate Coffee Milk	Iced Tea/Lemon Wedges Milk	Coffee Milk
"A" Watch - Mr. Johnson	**Wednesday 9 Feb. - Mr. Johnson**	**"B" Watch - Mr. Duvall**
Apple Juice 8oz. 120C	Beef Vegetable Soup 1c. 163C	Chopped Sirloin 600C
Assorted Cereal	Saltine Crackers/White Bread	Smothered Onion
Hot Cream of Wheat 1c. 133C	USNA Club Sandwich W/Turkey 420C	Parsleyed Potatoes ½c. 120C
Fresh Oranges	Ham and Bacon	Mixed Vegetables 45C
Scrambled Eggs ½c. 100C	Sliced American Cheese	Lettuce/Tomato/Cucumber Salad
Broiled Bacon 1sl. 45C	Sliced Lettuce/Tomato/Onion	French/Caesar's Dressing
Plain Toast Butter	Mayonnaise PCS Potato Chips	White Bread Butter
Honey Dipped Donuts	Marble Sheet Cake 350C	Vanilla Ice Cream W/Asstd Topping
Hot Chocolate Coffee Milk	Lemonade Milk	Coffee Milk
"A" Watch - Mr. Johnson	**Thursday 10 Feb. - Mr. Johnson**	**"B" Watch - Mr. Duvall**
Orange Juice 8oz. 120C	Chicken Noodle Soup 1c. 130C	Beef Stroganoff ½c. 400C
Assorted Cereal	Saltine Crackers	Egg Noodles ½c. 120C
Hot Grits ½c. 120C	French Bread Pizza ea. 450C	Lyonnaise Green Beans ½c. 45C
Fresh Bananas	Doritos	Chef's Salad 100C
Ham & Cheese Omelet	Antipasto Salad ½c. 110C	Russian Dressing
Lyonnaise Potatoes	Italian Dressing	Italian Dressing
Plain Toast Butter	Specky Vanilla Ice Cream	White Bread Butter
Hot Chocolate Coffee Milk	Sugar Cones	Apple Pie 1/6sl. 410C
	Orangeade Milk	Coffee Milk
"A" Watch - Mr. Johnson	**Friday 11 Feb. - Mr. Johnson**	**"B" Watch - Mr. Tubaya**
Orange Juice 8oz. 120C	French Onion Soup 1c. 132C	Seafood Dinner AvSv 700C
Assorted Cereal	Saltine Crackers	Macaroni and Cheese ½c. 235C
Hot Oatmeal 1c. 130C	El Rancho Stew 1c. 400C	Seasoned Spinach ½c. 60C
Fresh Bananas	Steamed Rice ½c. 120C	Tartar Sauce/Cocktail Sauce
Hot Cakes each 120C	Green Leafy Salad 10C	Cole Slaw W/Cream Dressing 85C
Ham Slices 100C	Ranch House/Caesar's Dressing	White Bread Butter
Maple Syrup Butter	Hot Biscuits Butter Honey	Chocolate Brownies 350C
Hot Chocolate Coffee Milk	Cannon Balls	Hot Tea/Lemon Wedges Milk
	Iced Tea/Lemon Wedges Milk	

In view of the average individual's dietary needs the Naval Academy menu looks high in calories. Just how many calories does the average midshipman eat? Do midshipmen get fat? These and other questions will be answered and discussed in the chapter on weight management.

NUTRITION GUIDELINES FOR ATHLETES

In summing up nutrition advice for athletes, Robert Serfass[8] wrote:

> Food and nutrient supplements to a well-balanced diet should be discouraged unless there is a clinical diagnosis of deficiency, because there is little evidence that such practice would improve performance.

Athletes are continually searching for a competitive edge over their opponents. Except for an occasional report of athletes using dangerous ergogenic aids, many athletes have resorted to nutrition supplements. Many wrongly assume that because proteins and vitamins (two overused supplements) are essential nutrients, extra amounts might be beneficial, but certainly not harmful.

The use of these relatively unproven ways to increase athletic performance continues because athletes and coaches are often misinformed about nutrition. They therefore become vulnerable to commercial sales pitches and promises of heightened performance by the supplement vendors. When the product is promoted by a paid celebrity athlete, the young athlete who identifies with the role model follows suit and uses the "magic potion."

Although food and nutrient supplements may not be beneficial and could be harmful, the caloric requirements for the athlete are important and should vary according to body size, age, type of competition and level of training. In addition, Serfass would advise the following:

- A diet distribution of 15% protein, 30% fat and 55% carbohydrate.
- Carbohydrate intake increase several days prior to competitive events requiring high glycogen stores, such as long distance running, swimming or cycling.
- Protein consumption is already high in the typical American diet, and an increase before an event may lower performance rather than enhance it.
- Except for an iron supplement, if warranted for females and teenage boys, vitamin supplements are not generally necessary or advised.

- Adequate water intake to prevent dehydration should be a primary consideration of every athlete during strenuous workouts or competition.
- Light pregame meals should be eaten approximately three hours prior to a contest. Carbohydrate intake within 1.5 and 2.0 hours of a contest may produce a transient hypoglycemia condition and a subsequent loss of energy.

In retrospect athletes must pay close attention to their diets, since poor nutrition may result in lowered performance. Good nutrition generally means having a diet adequately balanced in nutrients and calories while avoiding nutrient deficiencies. The well-nourished athlete need not add unnecessary and sometimes detrimental supplements to a diet to achieve full athletic potential.

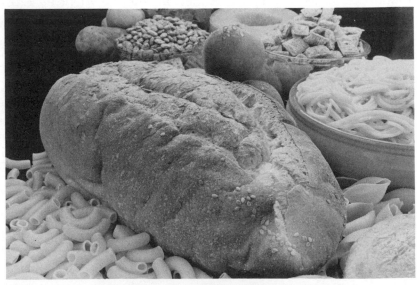

Good nutrition generally means having a diet adequately balanced in nutrients and calories while avoiding nutrient deficiencies. (David Madison photo)

REFERENCES

1. McArdle, William D., Frank I. Katch and Victor L. Katch, *Exercise Physiology: Energy, Nutrition, and Human Performance.* Philadelphia: Lea & Febiger, 1981.

2. Sharkey, Brian, *Physiology of Fitness.* Champaign, Ill.: Human Kinetics Publishers, 1979, p. 101.

3. Ibid, p. 271.

4. Cooper, Kenneth, *The Aerobics Program for Total Well-Being.* New York: M. Evans and Company, Inc., 1982, p. 38.

5. U.S. Department of Agriculture, *Nutrition and Your Health: Dietary Guidelines for Americans.* Washington D.C.: U.S. Government Printing Office, Home and Garden Bulletin No. 232.

6. Cooper, Kenneth, op. cit., pp. 81-96.

7. Dusek, Dorothy E., *Thin and Fit: Your Personal Lifestyle.* Belmont, CA.: Wadsworth Publishing Company, 1982, p. 146.

8. Serfass, Robert C., "Nutrition for the Athlete Update, 1982." *Contemporary Nutrition,* Vol. 7, No. 4, April, 1982.

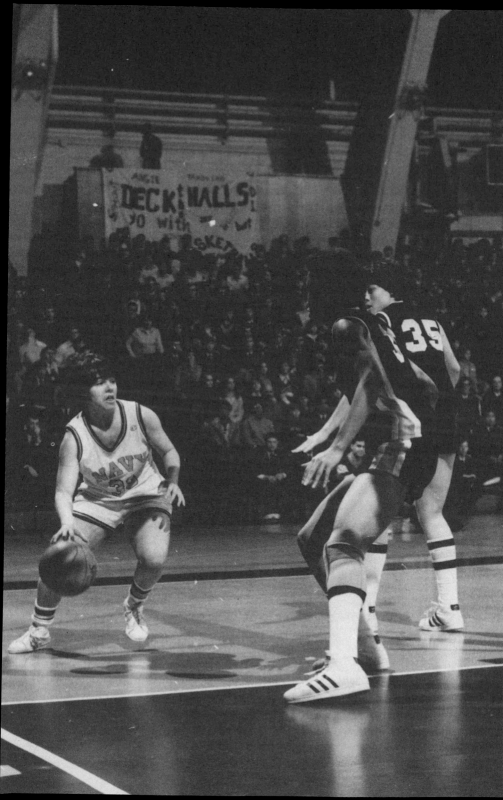

WEIGHT REDUCTION AND FITNESS

The struggle against this slowly
advancing glacier of lard begins
before we attain our majority.
Dr. George Sheehan
Dr. Sheehan on Running

OBJECTIVES

- Describe use of height/weight charts to determine body weight.
- Explain use of the Mahoney formula to determine body weight.
- Explain importance of measuring body fat.
- Describe how overfatness relates to exercise and health.
- Discuss the relationship between calories, metabolism and weight control.
- Identify several factors which cause us to gain excess fat.
- Describe how a proper diet helps maintain desirable weight.

WHAT SHOULD I WEIGH?

When a person asks, "What should I weigh?" it is often really a way of asking, "Do you like the way I look? Am I too heavy or too thin?" If someone tells us that we should gain or lose some weight, we often respond that we would look just awful if we gained or lost *that* much weight.

Although most of us are more concerned about how we want to look than about what we should weigh, in this chapter we will concentrate on your ideal weight. Interestingly, when you weigh what you should, you almost always like the way you look.

Height and weight charts

The typical way for an adult to determine proper body weight is to consult a height and weight chart. A range of weight is indicated for your height and body frame (small, medium or large). If your weight falls within the range for your height and body frame, you are considered to be "normal" for your age.

Most height and weight charts have been developed by insurance companies. They are based on actuarial data and not revised very often. The most popular chart is the one published by the Metropolitan Life Insurance Company. It is designed mainly for men and women over twenty-five years of age.

The weight variance for selected heights ranges from twenty to forty pounds on many charts. The range for a five-foot-tall woman, for example, is twenty-nine pounds. On the men's chart, the range is thirty-five pounds for a five-foot ten-inch man. Because the charts are designed for average adults, there are individuals who do not fall within the chart ranges. Football players or body builders with high levels of lean body weight and low body fat might well exceed the upper range. Competitive marathoners might also be far below the bottom range because of low fat levels. Such charts, therefore, have limited value in answering the question of how much you should weigh to be healthy.

Height and weight standards for midshipmen

Certain occupations may have height and weight restrictions because of safety or sports rules. Other occupations may establish height and weight standards to conform to image or appearance requirements inherent in the work.

For example, military personnel, police officers, jockeys, models and linebackers on professional football teams have to meet height and weight standards as occupational specifications rather than for reasons of health. In some instances these standards rule out persons who are overfat.

Height and weight standards are part of the medical considerations for admission to the U.S. Naval Academy and are expressed as minimal and maximal weights for specific heights in men and women. In special and unusual circumstances waivers are granted to candidates, but the charts clearly indicate that a wide allowance of weight exists in specific height categories. For example, five-foot ten-inch men could vary from 123 pounds to 215 pounds—a difference of nintey-two pounds.

WEIGHT STANDARDS (Men)

Height*	62	63	64	65	66	67	68	69	70	71	72	73	74	75	76	77	78
Weight:																	
Minimum	103	104	105	106	107	111	115	119	123	127	131	135	139	143	147	151	153
Maximum	168	174	179	186	191	197	203	209	215	221	227	233	240	246	253	260	267

WEIGHT STANDARDS (Women)

Height*	60	61	62	63	64	65	66	67	68	69	70	71	72	73	74	75	76	77	78
Weight:																			
Minimum	94	96	98	100	102	104	106	109	112	115	118	122	125	128	132	136	139	143	147
Maximum	125	127	130	134	138	142	147	151	156	160	165	170	175	180	184	189	195	200	205

*Waiver for height up to 80 inches may be granted to a limited number of candidates with exceptional scholastic leadership achievement.

The Mahoney formula
Another often used method to estimate body weight is the Mahoney formula. Theoretically the formula estimates an "idealized" weight of a person with a medium build at a specific height. Here is how you calculate it:

MEN	WOMEN
Height (in.)	Height (in.)
× 4.0	× 3.5
Sub totl	Sub totl
− 130	− 110
Ideal Body Weight	Ideal Body Weight

Using this formula, a 5′ 10″ male with a medium body build would weigh 150 pounds. A 5′ 0″ female would weight 100 pounds. Cooper uses this formula, but for men he subtracts 128 from the subtotal rather than 130, and for women 108 rather than 110. He also increases the ideal weight for individuals with large body frames by 102.

By multiplying one's ideal weight by one of the following activity level numbers, one can also estimate the number of calories which should be consumed on an average daily basis.

13   very inactive
14   slightly inactive
15   moderately active
16   relatively active
17   frequently, strenuously active

Body composition and the charts

The wide range of weights within each height category of the charts allows for large variations in body fat, muscle weight and bone density, and these are the important factors when considering the health and fitness of each individual.

Perhaps the major focus today is upon the factor of overfatness. Known as obesity, an excessive amount of body fat is a legitimate health concern because of its relationship to several degenerative disorders. With respect to physical fitness, excessive amounts of body fat generally lower one's ability to do aerobic exercise—and often, because aerobic exercises are more strenuous for the obese person, these individuals tend to avoid this beneficial type of exercise.

While height and weight charts serve the useful purpose of screening large groups of people, more accurate measures of body composition are available. On an individual basis, the diet- and fitness-conscious person should seek these alternative methods to get a more accurate picture of body fat, and more and more people who desire more precise measures of body composition are now doing so because they are more readily available.

As weight management is discussed more fully in this chapter, it is important to remember that the concept of *overweight* is mainly a subjective self-image concern whereas the concept of *overfat* is a more objective concern about health. We shall therefore focus our attention on overfatness.

MEASURING BODY FAT

No measuring device is absolutely perfect for estimating body fat, but there are several reliable indirect methods which take into account the fat content as well as the lean body weight of the individual. Lean body weight is an estimate of your percent body weight minus all stored fat. This measure is important for those on a strict diet and for athletes who are aiming for a specific body weight and percent of body fat.

Many university research laboratories use a hydrostatic (underwater) weighing technique, a method designed to measure the individual's body density or specific gravity. Body density is the ratio of a person's weight in air to the person's weight when submerged in water. The percent of body fat is then calculated from the known body density.

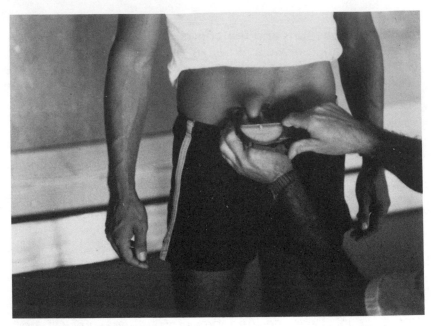

Abdominal Skin Fold Test

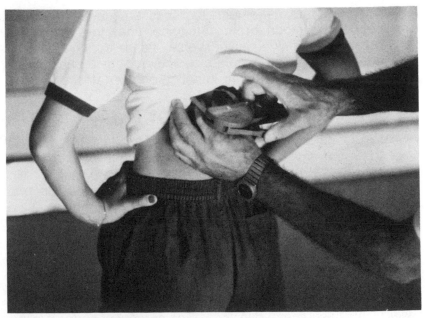

Subscapular Skin Fold Test

Your Current Body Composition and Ideal Weight·

Step 1 LBW (lean body weight):

Women:
20.20

+_____ = (.635 × your weight in pounds)
_____ = a subtotal of above
-_____ = (.503 × your subscapular skin-
          fold, in mm.)
_____ = LBW

Men:
22.62

+_____ = (.793 × your weight in pounds)
_____ = a subtotal of above
-_____ = (.801 × your abdominal skin-
          fold, in mm.)
_____ = LBW

Step 2% Fat:

For Women and Men:

$$\frac{\text{Body Weight - LBW}}{\text{Body Weight}} \times 100 = \underline{\hspace{1cm}} \text{ Current \% Fat}$$

Categories:

Women					Men
30%	( )	Obesity	( )		20%
25%	( )	Overweight	( )		15%
22-20%	( )	Ideal	( )		12½-10%
Below 20%	( )	Underfat	( )		Below 10%

Step 3 Relative Weights for You:

Women:			Men:
$\frac{\text{LBW}}{.70}$	=	Your "Obesity" Weight =	$\frac{\text{LBW}}{.80}$
$\frac{\text{LBW}}{.75}$	=	Your "Overweight" Weight =	$\frac{\text{LBW}}{.85}$
$\frac{\text{LBW}}{.78}$	=	Your "High Ideal" Weight =	$\frac{\text{LBW}}{.875}$
$\frac{\text{LBW}}{.80}$	=	Your "Low Ideal" Weight =	$\frac{\text{LBW}}{.90}$
Below The Above Figure	=	Your "Underfat" Weight =	Below The Above Figure

*Wilmore, Jack, Ph.D. Director, Department of Physical Education, Exercise and Sport Sciences Laboratory McKale Memorial Center, The University of Arizona, Tucson, Arizona 85721.

Because hydrostatic weighing requires special facilities and special calculations, various skinfold techniques have been developed to estimate percent of body fat. These techniques are relatively simple to apply and can be easily administered to large groups of individuals. For general population screening they provide good estimates of an individual's body fat. The theory behind the use of skinfold techniques is that most of the body's fat storage areas lie directly beneath the skin.

Generally reliable measures of body fat are obtained using the skinfold technique when 1) the tester is trained and experienced in taking skinfold measurements, and 2) a good instrument such as the Lange skinfold caliper is used.

Researchers have worked on skinfold measures for many years attempting to develop an accurate and reliable test to estimate body fat. A recent test developed by Wilmore consists of taking only one skinfold measure on men and one on women. From this single measure the individual's lean body weight and percent of fat can be estimated. Wilmore's test procedure is simple to administer, simple to calculate and permits testing of many people in a very short period of time. In addition the procedure allows one to calculate actual body weight at hypothetical percentages of fat. This therefore helps the person determine how much weight (fat) must be lost to reach the ideal or desired weight level.

Overfat and underfat
The human body has the capacity to store widely varying amounts of body fat. Marathon runners often carry as little as 4-6% fat, whereas sumo wrestlers may well exceed 50%. There is, however, a percentage of body fat which represents the desirable or healthy range for most individuals, and estimates are that this range falls somewhere between ten and twenty percent. This level takes into account fat which is essential for proper body functioning such as storage of energy, protection of other body tissue and organs and production of various body secretions.

Researchers may differ somewhat about the precise limits of the normal and desirable percent of body fat ranges. But virtually all would agree that too little or too much fat can adversely affect health. Anorexia nervosa, which results in excessive thinness, has become a serious health disorder, especially among young teenage females. On the other hand, excess fat is perhaps a more serious health problem for the general population. Our general focus in this chapter is on excess fat and how an individual can effectively reach and maintain a desirable body weight.

The concern about Americans becoming overfat is not a recent one. In 1969 a Metropolitan Life Insurance Company brochure stated the following:

> Excess poundage puts undue strain on the human body. People who are overweight seem to be more susceptible to certain diseases, especially heart and circulatory diseases, and diabetes. They may have less resistance to infection, notably from pneumonia and influenza. Indications are that they suffer from other illnesses, such as gallbladder and liver disorders, to a greater degree than slim people. They even tend to have more accidents.

Body fat averages for men and women

Estimates of the percentage of body fat among American population groups tend to differ somewhat from study to study. Most studies indicate that young male college students average about 15-16 percent fat and young college females about 20-21 percent. Some studies report female averages as high as 25-26 percent. Because of anatomical and physiological differences, females consistently average 5-6 percent more body fat than males.

What is most alarming to the medical community is that these percentages tend to rise as American men and women get older. It is well documented that although most Americans become less active as they get older, they rarely change their eating patterns to reduce caloric intake. Estimates are that middle-aged men and women in the United States have gradually increased body fat by as much as 10-20 percent by the time they reach forty years of age. More often than not, most individuals do not notice this gradual increase in weight (mostly fat), or else they tend to assume it is somehow "natural," since they often think they eat less than they used to.

How do individuals know when they are overfat? McArdle, Katch and Katch say that this point is reached when women exceed 30% fat and men 20%. Cooper suggests that when either men or women exceed 20% body fat regardless of age, they have become overfat. For those interested in good health and fitness, the 20% estimate is safe and desirable as the upper limit of fat.

And one further word about personal "guesstimates": Using the mirror to estimate your percentage of body fat, and casual observation of your eating habits, are poor ways to achieve reliable measures. Most of us rationalize too much about our fat and our eating habits, believing we eat fewer calories than we actually do, and underestimating our percent of body fat—which causes us to give all kinds of erroneous reasons for our weight gains. The best advice is to be truthful with yourself and get an accurate assessment of your percent of body fat and of the actual number of calories consumed on a daily basis. When you do this you will be taking the first positive step toward improved health and fitness.

CALORIES AND BODY FAT

Calories and metabolism A calorie is defined as the amount of energy required to raise one liter of water one degree centigrade. Simply stated, a calorie is a measure of energy calculated from the amount of heat generated. With few exceptions, each morsel of food eaten by each of us contains energy which is locked in its molecular structure. Different types of food have molecules which have varying amounts of calories. Fats, for example, contain more calories per gram than do carbohydrates or proteins.

The word "metabolism" is often used in discussions of calories. The term refers to the process whereby the body's cells oxidize food materials and release energy for physiological work. The term "metabolic rate" refers to the rate at which energy is released from foods. At rest, for example, an individual may have a metabolic rate of 60 to 70 calories per hour. During strenuous activity this rate might increase to 200 or 300 calories per hour.

Many factors influence metabolic rate. Age, thyroid gland secretion, body temperature, intensity of activity and the content of meals are just a few of these factors. These individual variations make comparisons between people somewhat difficult.

The basal metabolic rate is a measurement that makes comparisons less burdensome. The standard procedure for determining this requires certain restrictions, such as 1) complete mental rest, 2) no exercise for 30 minutes to an hour before the test; 3) no food intake within the past 12 hours; and 4) comfortable air temperature during the test. Under these

Table 3.3 Calories Burned per Quarter-Hour, per Hour and per Day According to Weight

Weight*	Cal./Hour	Cal./Day	Cal./¼ Hr.	Weight*	Cal./Hour	Cal./Day	Cal./¼ Hr.	Weight*	Cal./Hour	Cal./Day	Cal./¼ Hr.
75	34.4625	827.1	8.62	114	52.383	1257.19	13.10	153	70.3035	1687.28	17.58
76	34.922	838.128	8.73	115	52.8425	1268.22	13.21	154	70.763	1698.31	17.69
77	35.3815	849.156	8.85	116	53.302	1279.25	13.33	155	71.2225	1709.34	17.80
78	35.841	860.184	8.96	117	53.7615	1290.28	13.44	156	71.682	1720.37	17.92
79	36.3005	871.212	9.08	118	54.221	1301.3	13.55	157	72.1415	1731.4	18.04
80	36.76	882.24	9.19	119	54.6805	1312.33	13.67	158	72.601	1742.42	18.15
81	37.2195	893.268	9.30	120	55.14	1323.36	13.77	159	73.0605	1753.45	18.27
82	37.679	904.296	9.42	121	55.5995	1334.39	13.90	160	73.52	1764.48	18.38
83	38.1385	915.324	9.54	122	56.059	1345.42	14.01	161	73.9795	1775.51	18.50
84	38.598	926.352	9.65	123	56.5185	1356.44	14.13	162	74.439	1786.54	18.61
85	39.0575	937.38	9.76	124	56.978	1367.47	14.24	163	74.8985	1797.56	18.73
86	39.517	948.408	9.88	125	57.4375	1378.5	14.36	164	75.358	1808.59	18.84
87	39.9765	959.436	9.99	126	57.897	1389.53	14.47	165	75.8175	1819.62	18.95
88	40.436	970.464	10.11	127	58.3565	1400.56	14.59	166	76.277	1830.65	19.07
89	40.8955	981.492	10.22	128	58.816	1411.58	14.70	167	76.7365	1841.68	19.18
90	41.355	992.52	10.34	129	59.2755	1422.61	14.82	168	77.196	1852.7	19.30
91	41.8145	1003.55	10.45	130	59.735	1433.64	14.93	169	77.6655	1863.73	19.41
92	42.274	1014.58	10.57	131	60.1945	1444.67	15.05	170	78.115	1874.76	19.53
93	42.7335	1025.6	10.68	132	60.654	1455.7	15.16	171	78.5745	1885.79	19.64
94	43.193	1036.63	10.80	133	61.1135	1466.72	15.28	172	79.034	1896.82	19.76
95	43.6525	1047.66	10.91	134	61.573	1477.75	15.39	173	79.4935	1907.84	19.87
96	44.112	1058.69	11.02	135	62.0325	1488.78	15.50	174	79.953	1918.87	19.99
97	44.5715	1069.72	11.14	136	62.492	1499.81	15.62	175	80.4125	1929.9	20.10
98	45.031	1080.74	11.26	137	62.9515	1510.84	15.74	176	80.872	1940.93	20.22
99	45.4905	1091.77	11.37	138	63.411	1521.86	15.85	177	81.3315	1951.96	20.33
100	45.95	1102.8	11.49	139	63.8705	1532.89	15.97	178	81.791	1962.98	20.45
101	46.4095	1113.83	11.60	140	64.33	1543.92	16.08	179	82.2505	1974.01	20.56
102	46.869	1124.86	11.72	141	64.7895	1554.95	16.20	180	82.71	1985.04	20.68
103	47.3285	1135.88	11.83	142	65.249	1566.98	16.31	181	83.1695	1996.07	20.79
104	47.788	1146.91	11.95	143	65.7085	1577	16.43	182	83.629	2007.1	20.91
105	48.2475	1157.94	12.06	144	66.168	1588.03	16.54	183	84.0885	2018.12	21.02

Table 3.3 Calories Burned per Quarter-Hour, per Hour and per Day According to Weight

Weight*	Cal./Hour	Cal./Day	Cal./¼ Hr.	Weight*	Cal./Hour	Cal./Day	Cal./¼ Hr.	Weight*	Cal./Hour	Cal./Day	Cal./¼ Hr.
106	48.707	1168.97	12.18	145	66.6275	1599.06	16.66	184	84.548	2029.15	21.14
107	49.1665	1180	12.29	146	67.087	1610.09	16.77	185	85.0075	2040.18	21.25
108	49.626	1191.02	12.40	147	67.5465	1621.12	16.89	186	85.467	2051.21	21.37
109	50.0855	1202.05	12.52	148	68.006	1632.14	17.00	187	85.9265	2062.24	21.48
110	50.545	1213.08	12.64	149	68.4655	1643.17	17.11	188	86.386	2073.26	21.60
111	51.0045	1224.11	12.75	150	68.925	1654.2	17.24	189	86.8455	2084.29	21.71
112	51.464	1235.14	12.87	151	69.3845	1665.23	17.35	190	87.305	2095.32	21.83
113	51.9235	1246.16	12.98	152	69.844	1676.26	17.46	191†	87.7645	2106.35	21.94

*Weight is given in pounds.
†If your weight is more than 191 pounds, divide it by 2, find that weight on the chart, and then double the calorie figure.

From *Thin and Fit: Your Personal Lifestyle* by Dorothy E. Dusek. Belmont, CA., Wadsworth Publishing Co., 1982. Used by permission.

conditions a person's lowest wakeful level of burning calories is ascertained.

It is apparent from the above discussion that metabolism and calories are inextricably associated with fluctuations in body weight. Any assessment of our caloric intake and output must therefore take into consideration our metabolic rate.

Fat storage Many of us have contempt for the fat that results in undesirable bulges in the wrong places on our bodies—we wish it would rearrange itself to conform to our ideal self-image. But unfortunately our bodies rarely comply with our desire, and the fat keeps piling up in the wrong places. Soon we either accept this as inevitable or take the only course of action available to us — lower the total amount of fat on our bodies and thus cause many of the bulges to disappear.

We are wise to have contempt for excessive fat and should be highly motivated to leave the extra calories on the grocery store shelves. But we must also appreciate and respect our body's unique ability to store fat. Think about it. The body's fat storage system was designed to save unused fuel and store it as a high-octane source of energy for emergencies. In the animal world, migratory birds eat more and accumulate fat under their wings for long flights, which enables them to travel nonstop to their destinations.

Remember that all food substances, when eaten in excess, can be converted to fat and stored in fat cells. By simply enlarging themselves, these cells in adults store this high-potency fuel. When these stores of fats are needed, the body breaks them down into usable components (fatty acids) and releases them into the bloodstream. Because each gram of fat contains approximately 9.0 calories, while carbohydrates and proteins contain about half that value, you can readily see that the body has designed a remarkable system to store energy.

Fat is our physiological friend and only becomes unfriendly and harmful when we become over-indulgent in our food consumption.

The calorie game The process by which we gain and lose weight is relatively simple. When we expend more calories than we consume, we lose weight. When we consume more calories than we expend, we gain weight.

Monitoring caloric input and output is a somewhat more complex process. For most individuals it is also tedious and boring. Factors which must be taken into account include body weight, age and metabolic rate. In addition, all food eaten, along with each type of activity (recorded every quarter-hour), must be catalogued daily. When you combine these record-keeping chores with intense motivation and discipline to alter eating behaviors, you will be able to control your body weight effectively.

Fortunately many individuals intuitively regulate caloric input and output, thereby maintaining a desirable and stable body weight. The rest of us who overconsume the "fruits of the good life" must direct our efforts toward managing these dietary variables if we expect to achieve a desirable and healthful weight level. Unfortunately the most difficult part of the process is changing eating behaviors which have become well-ingrained habits.

Those who play and *win* the calorie game usually have excellent social support from family, friends or others in an organized program. As you play the game, also keep several other factors in mind:

Input factors
- All foods contain calories and therefore can be stored as body fat.
- One pound of body fat is equivalent to 3500 calories. To lose a pound of fat (usually done at the rate of 1-2 a week), you must expend 3500 more calories than you consume.

Output factors
- Your base level of daily caloric expenditure depends upon your weight and age (check the charts for these numbers).
- Caloric expenditures increase when you exercise more (a five-mile walk at a 20-minute per mile pace burns almost 200 calories).

WHY WE GAIN WEIGHT

America truly is the land of milk and honey. Walk any American ocean beach on a typical summer Sunday afternoon and you will easily observe the milk and honey bulging from the midriffs, thighs, arms, legs and faces of our adult population.

Is obesity a self-inflicted health disorder caused simply by human behavior known as overeating? Have we reached such a plateau in our economic and social development where we now "live to eat" rather than "eat to live?" Why do we overeat? Let us examine some of the reasons.

Physical inactivity In America, where increased mechanization has produced a less active society, the reduced level of human energy expenditure certainly has influenced the overweight problem. An adipose deposition cycle begins as people become generally less active. As they become less active they get fatter. To complete the cycle—as they get fatter they once again have less energy and become more inactive. The cycle repeats itself over and over as the fat gradually becomes more visible creeping in beneath our skin.

There is another factor to consider about physical activity and weight regulation. On a short-term basis activity seems to have an insignificant effect on caloric expenditure. For example, since one pound of fat equals 3500 calories, a 120-pound woman would have to run about 48 miles for nearly six consecutive hours to burn one pound of fat. But in the long term consider the following. That same woman could run one mile a day and lose one pound of fat in 48 days without reducing her caloric intake — in one year she could lose eight pounds *without dieting.*

Because physical inactivity has contributed to our adult obesity problem, physical activity will certainly help solve it.

The genetic factor In August 1981 Gilbert B. Forbes[7] summarized some of the research directed at the question of whether obesity was a genetic disease. Although Forbes does not define the threshold or limits of obesity, he does conclude that the available evidence indicates that the tendency toward obesity is inherited and that the genes responsible find expression through the abundance of modern food. He further reports that studies indicate obese individuals do eat in excess of physiological need and have very sedentary lifestyles. This suggests that the environmental factors also play an essential role in the obesity process.

Direct intervention and management of obesity is possible and desirable for individuals who may have a genetic tendency to the disorder. A distinction must be made between hunger and appetite, however. Hunger is a physiological phenomenon; appetite has a psychological foundation. It is generally thought that persons with a genetic obesity condition have a faulty appetite mechanism rather than a faulty hunger mechanism. Our appetite often overrides our hunger drive whenever there is an abundant supply of food available to us.

Psycho-social influences Eating behaviors in the U.S. are closely linked with our psychological and social development as children. Food often serves as a pacifier, a reward and a connector with special events in our lives. Parents use food to reward good behavior. Food is often withheld to punish poor behavior. Food (especially the high-calorie sort) is used to celebrate birthdays, athletic and performing achievements and good grades.

For most of us food is associated with positive, warm and relaxed feelings. It is therefore easily understood why we often eat when we are tense, feel unloved, frustrated, bored or otherwise stressed.

Unfortunately these associated behaviors also cause us to gain weight although this weight gain often occurs so slowly that we hardly notice it happening.

Socio-cultural influences America, the great melting pot, has absorbed many different people with varied cultural backgrounds from everywhere in the world. With these immigrants came a heterogeneous pool of social, religious and ethnic customs, and many groups brought distinct culinary preferences and eating traditions.

Eating simply to stay alive and healthy relegates food to something mundane in our lives. Food has far greater implications, but many of our traditional habits and associations with food have contributed to our obesity dilemma.

Many of us who eat at our customary family and social gatherings do so because it is socially accepted and socially expected. How many of us consciously regulate our food intake at lower levels at other meals on days of these occasions? If we were able to regulate our intake better to balance the level of expenditure, most of us could maintain a desirable weight level. This requires careful planning and a disciplined will.

HOW WE LOSE WEIGHT

Following careful assessment of your percentage of body fat, you might decide to begin a weight reduction program. If you do not exceed the 30% (women) or the 20% (men) level and want to lose a few pounds, you might establish your own individual program. If you exceed these levels, a consultation with your physician might be a prudent and sensible way to begin. If you exceed 39% fat, this is considered clinical obesity and medical guidance is strongly advised.

There are many popular diet programs available to the public. But what criteria should you use to determine if the program will benefit you. The first and most important question is whether the program is safe. If the program causes additional health risk, you may want to discard it or work closely with your doctor. Secondly, will the program realistically help you reach the goals you have established for yourself.? Thirdly, do you have the willpower, discipline and motivation to carry through with the program? If you cannot honestly answer these three questions in the affirmative, you may not be ready to embark on a serious weight reduction program.

From a health viewpoint there are several other factors which you may wish to consider:

1) Will my program contain all nutrients in the appropriate amounts and correct proportions for maintaining good health? Obtaining all nutrients may be difficult on a diet of less than 1000-1200 calories a day.

2) Will my program severely restrict the intake of certain nutrients such as carbohydrates, fats or proteins? Severe restrictions of any single nutrient may be risky. Your program should therefore focus on reducing caloric intake, not on reducing nutrient intake.

3) Will my program severely restrict or eliminate foods which are the most nutritious foods among my favorites? As in any normal diet, eating a variety of foods makes dining a pleasure and will keep you motivated to stay on your program.

4) Will my program include a gradual increase in my level of physical activity? Exercising along with dieting helps lose pounds fast and also prevents the body from losing lean body weight (muscle tissue) along with body fat.

5) Will my program be supported by my friends or relatives, or do these close associates of mine tend to sabotage weight-reduction programs? Social support is important for your morale and dedication in achieving your goal. If this support is not readily available, you may have to seek it in another type of support group, such as a weight-control or exercise class.

6) Will my program include weekly goals and an effective and efficient way to track my progress with good record-keeping? Setting goals and monitoring progress closely is a good motivator, but remember that 1-2 pounds a week weight loss should be maximum.

Diet options Within the parameters established above, you have three general options in adopting a weight-loss program. These are:

A. Expend more energy and maintain caloric intake
B. Maintain energy level and reduce caloric intake
C. Expend more energy and reduce caloric intake

For many of the reasons alluded to in the foregoing discussion Dusek[8] highly recommends option C. Options A and B according to Dusek have high failure rates.

Popular diets Commercially published books, newspapers, popular self-improvement magazines and even TV advertising extol the virtues of new diet formulas, plans and programs. Many diet books have become best-sellers. What special allure do these programs have for the public? Are chronic dieters in any way justified in believing that the next new best-selling diet might end all diets?

The serious, non-obese, but overfat, dieter should carefully evaluate the merits of any dietary program regardless of the slick sales pitches or celebrity appeal often identified with the diet. And an obese individual should work closely with a physician before choosing any of the popular weight-reduction programs.

The alert and informed dieter should recognize popular diets which can be dangerous to health regardless of the promised short-term results. Any popular diet which prohibits the intake of any of the major food sources (carbohydrates, proteins or fats) should be viewed with extreme caution. Popular diets which allow you only to drink or eat the company's own special concoctions (even though many contain vitamin supplementation) should be evaluated carefully. Also, watch out for diet programs that promise to share their "secret formula" with you.

There are no secret formulas when one desires to lose body fat. Keep a balanced diet, reduce caloric intake and exercise moderately, and you will lose weight. The major obstacle to successful weight control is not lack of knowledge; it is your attitude and your ability to control eating behaviors effectively.

Since most quick diet schemes do not work—mainly because most dieters are seeking rapid weight loss without the supporting behavioral changes—evaluating a diet program is an important step in successful, permanent weight reduction. Unfortunately most "popular" diet books and programs do not effectively deal with long-range behavioral change strategies. Neither do many discuss the more important nutritional information. Instead, most entertain us with lively personal testimonials or exotic unproven eating theories.

Before investing in any diet program, measure its merits against a few of the following criteria:

1. Does the program discuss the importance of nutrients, such as carbohydrates, fats, proteins, vitamins, minerals and water? What percentage of daily intake of these substances is recommended? **Programs should not severely restrict or alter the normal daily recommendations.**

2. What does the program indicate about caloric restrictions? **Programs which restrict total daily caloric intake below 1000 calories should be physician-approved.**

3. Does the program recommend eating a diversified and wholesome diet? Or does the program advocate special commercially produced or exotic foods which are costly and mainly benefit the manufacturer? **Dieters quickly lose interest in single-food diets or exotic diets.**

4. Does the program discuss eating behavior changes and provide personal or group strategies which require a long-range commitment and a permanent change in eating behavior?
Few diet programs succeed without such strategies and social support to maintain them.

5. Does the program provide information about how to measure your percentage of body fat or where you can obtain an assessment of it?
A program which does not address the body fat issue is sidestepping one of the most important health reasons for dieting — specifically the reduction of excess body fat.

6. Does the program require and/or provide a diet diary or other means of diet record-keeping?
A diary can be a key motivator in long-range success and it gives you a fairly accurate record of average caloric intake and expenditures.

7. With these six practical concerns, a good weight-reduction program must inspire you to initiate and stay with the program until your desired weight goals are reached

MIDSHIPMEN'S DIETS

Although there is no statistical evidence to prove it, estimates are that midshipmen average about the same levels of body fat at the time of induction at the Naval Academy as their college-bound high school classmates. For men this is between 15-20%; for women the average is 20-25%.

Food is nutritious and plentiful at the Naval Academy. The Food Services Officer reports that if midshipmen were to eat a normal helping of everything served at the three meals, they would consume 4,500 calories. Few do, but a lot of calories are available.

As a rule midshipmen in the fourth class, the plebes, do not gain weight. Some experience weight losses. Plebes are physically more active than men and women in the other three classes. They have not yet learned to manage their time efficiently. Plebes frequently rush out of the ward room at the very first opportunity because time is so precious a commodity.

DESIRABLE WEIGHTS FOR MEN AND WOMEN

According to Height and Frame, Ages 25 and Over

Height (in shoes)	Weight in Pounds (in Indoor Clothing) *		
	Small Frame	Medium Frame	Large Frame
MEN			
5' 2"	128-134	131-141	138-150
3"	130-136	133-143	140-153
4"	132-138	135-145	142-156
5"	134-140	137-148	144-160
6"	136-142	139-151	146-164
7"	138-145	142-154	149-168
8"	140-148	145-157	152-172
9"	142-151	148-160	155-176
10"	144-154	151-163	158-180
11"	146-157	154-166	161-184
6' 0"	149-160	157-170	164-188
1"	152-164	160-174	168-192
2"	155-168	164-178	172-197
3"	158-172	167-182	176-202
4"	162-176	171-187	181-207
WOMEN			
4'10"	102-111	109-121	118-131
11"	103-113	111-123	120-134
5' 0"	104-115	113-126	122-137
1"	106-118	115-129	125-140
2"	108-121	118-132	128-143
3"	111-124	121-135	131-147
4"	114-127	124-138	134-151
5"	117-130	127-141	137-155
6"	120-133	130-144	140-159
7"	123-136	133-147	143-163
8"	126-139	136-150	146-167
9"	129-142	139-153	149-170
10"	132-145	142-156	152-173
11"	135-148	145-159	155-176
6' 0"	138-151	148-162	158-179

* Indoor clothing weighing 3 lbs. for women and 5 lbs. for men
** Shoes with 1-inch heels

Source: 1979 Build Study; Society of Actuaries and Association of Life Insurance Medical Directors of America, 1980   Courtesy of the Metropolitan Insurance Company

Car privileges change throughout the four years. Plebes do not rate riding in cars; as second classmen they are allowed to have vehicles within two miles of the Academy. By the time midshipmen are in the first class, they are permitted to have their cars in the Yard.

All of these factors decrease the caloric expenditure of midshipmen as the four years pass. The result is an increase in body fat. The same conditions appear to take place at West Point.

Documented studies conducted at West Point, the U.S. Military Academy, suggest a significant increase in body fat among men and women cadets during their four years of training. How this affects the short-range fitness level of cadets, or whether this extends into adulthood, is not clear.

REFERENCES

1. Mahoney, Michael and Kathryn Mahoney, "How Much Should You Weigh?" *Psychology Today*, May 1978.
2. Cooper, Kenneth, *The Aerobics Program for Total Well-Being*. New York: M. Evans and Company, Inc., 1982, p. 71.
3. Wilmore Formula, presented in *Aerobic Dance: A Way To Fitness*, By Judy Kisselle and Karen Mazzeo. Englewood: Morton Publishing Co., p. 163-164.
4. Metropolitan Life Insurance Company, *Four Steps to Weight Control*, 1969.
5. McArdle, William D., Frank I. Katch and Victor L. Katch, *Exercise Physiology: Energy, Nutrition and Human Performance*. Philadelphia: Lea & Febiger, 1981, p. 406.
6. Cooper, Kenneth, *The Aerobics Program for Total Well-Being*. New York: M. Evans and Company, Inc., 1982, p. 71.
7. Forbes, Gilbert B., "Is Obesity a Genetic Disease?" *Contemporary Nutrition*, August 1981, Vol. 6 No. 8.
8. Dusek, Dorothy, *Thin and Fit: Your Personal Lifestyle*. Belmont, CA: Wadsworth Publishing Company, pp. 38-39.

Additional references

Brody, Jane, *Jane Brody's Nutrition Book*. New York: Norton & Co., 1981.

Hafen, Brent Q., *Nutrition, Food, and Weight Control*. Boston: Allyn and Bacon, Inc., 1981.

Kreutler, Patricia A., *Nutrition*. Englewood Cliffs, NJ: Prentice-Hall, 1980.

Kirschman, John D. (director), *Nutrition Search Inc*. New York: McGraw-Hill Book Co., 1975.

Life Science Library, *Food and Nutrition*. Alexandria, Va: Time-Life Books, 1980.

Mayer, Jean, *A Diet for Living*. New York: D. McKay Co., 1975.

Wickham, Sandy J., *Human Nutrition*. Bowie, MD: Robert J. Brady Co., 1982.

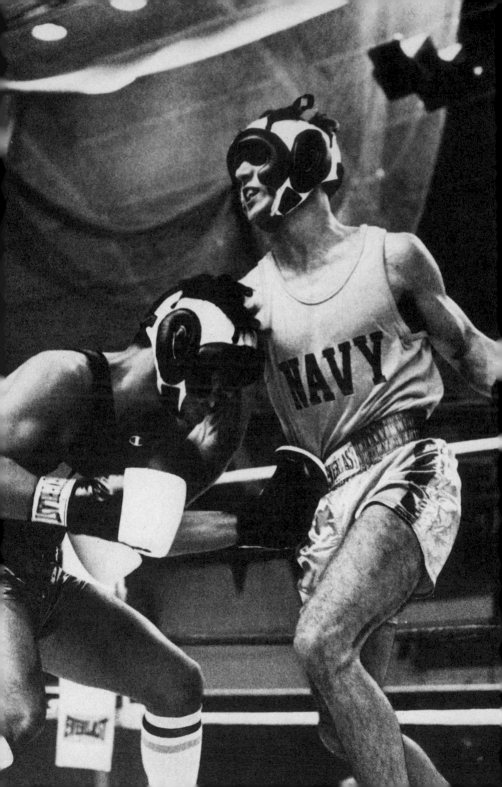

9

STRESS AND FITNESS

There have been challenges on and off the football field, and my ability to handle them has been dependent upon keeping everything in perspective.

Roger Staubach
Time Enough to Win

OBJECTIVES

- Define the term "stress."
- Discuss the positive and negative qualities of stress.
- Describe Selye's Stress Response.
- Identify stressors commonly experienced daily.
- Examine how stress may affect different individuals.
- List the signals of overstress.
- Describe Benson's Relaxation Response.
- Identify several methods of controlling stress.
- Discuss how midshipmen handle stress.

WHAT IS OVERSTRESS?

Butterflies fill your stomach before an important athletic contest. Your mind suddenly goes blank in the middle of a major exam. Your mouth feels like cotton as you rise to speak to a group of people. When you are frightened, your muscles instantly become tense. In these situations and in many others like them in daily life, you are experiencing temporary episodes of stress.

The noted endocrinologist Dr. Hans Selye[1] defined stress as the nonspecific response of the body to any demand made upon it. Selye, who pioneered much of the original research on stress, contends that the nonspecific response may be beneficial when pleasant (eustress) or harmful when unpleasant (distress).

Eustress Throughout our childhood we learn to expect certain body changes in situations of sudden and temporary stress. Most of us have learned to control the level of change and keep the stress-causing events in general perspective. We recognize that controlled stress helps us "key up" to improve our performance or enjoy our activities more. In this sense, the energy generated by internal stress is used for positive and constructive behaviors.

Distress But what happens to us when life becomes hectic and our pace quickens? Girdano and Everly state that stress is "...a fairly predictable arousal of psychophysiological (mind-body) systems which, if prolonged, can fatigue or damage the system to the point of malfunction and disease."[2]

Is it too much job stress that causes heart attacks in overworked middle-aged executives? Is the sedentary, deadline-conscious secretary who chain smokes over-stressed? Does the bored production-line worker take excessive sick days because of distress? Is stress out of control when the athlete or movie star takes drugs to get high? What types of pressures affect the parent who abuses a child, or the teenager who finds little to live for and commits suicide? In these regrettable cases, stress is undesirable and destructive.

The effects of long periods of stress can also be subtle, but experts tell us that too much psycho-social stress may lead to debilitating illnesses such as heart disease, ulcers and possibly cancer. Many of these disorders are self-inflicted, and we often lack the ability to view our attitudes as destructive. Barbara Brown describes stress as "...an unfavorable perception of the social environment and its dynamics."[3] Perhaps Alvin Toffler in *Future*

Shock[4] best explained how stress can have negative effects upon us. According to Toffler our inability to adapt to the accelerated rate of cultural and technological changes lies at the root of our stress.

STRESS AND WELLNESS

Simply acknowledging the desirable or the destructive qualities of stress indicates little about the intricate connection between stress and personal well-being. One must understand the concept of homeostasis, Selye's Stress Response Theory, the common stressors that elicit a stress response, the effects that stress has upon different types of individuals, the overstress signals, and the positive coping behaviors that can help us manage stress effectively.

Although Toffler and others might conclude that people in general have not yet learned to control modern stress, the human species has survived throughout history because of its successful adaptibility to change. As we continue to face the challenge of a rapidly changing technological world, we must remember that effective management of stress is just as important to our well-being as our diet and regular exercise program.

Homeostasis

As external and internal stimuli impact upon the human organism, the physiological equilibrium is temporarily altered. For example, when you exercise your internal temperature rises automatically. Because it could be dangerous if it gets too high, your body automatically causes you to perspire in an effort to cool you down. Hundreds of these miraculous adjustments take place in your body every minute of your life. If conditions push these delicate balances too far in either direction, the homeostasis is disrupted and the body loses its physiological integrity.

Under the usual and normal short episodes of stress, your homeostasis is temporarily out of balance and quickly returns to its normal state. However, in the absence of stimuli or when stimuli are too intense or come in frequent salvos, your body may lose its ability to maintain its internal equilibrium. Each of us easily recognizes this state of imbalance, which often shows up as pain, fatigue or sudden illness.

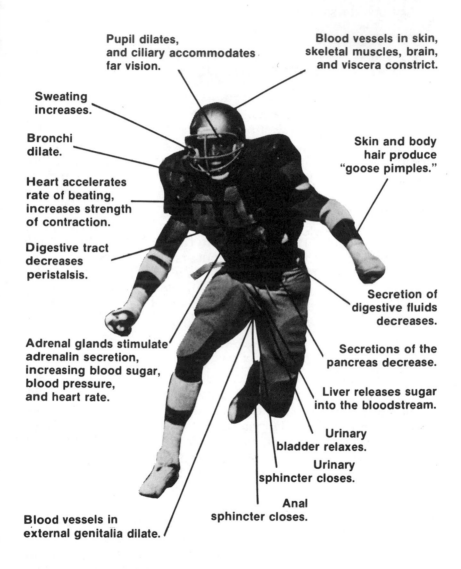

Pupil dilates, and ciliary accommodates far vision.

Blood vessels in skin, skeletal muscles, brain, and viscera constrict.

Sweating increases.

Bronchi dilate.

Skin and body hair produce "goose pimples."

Heart accelerates rate of beating, increases strength of contraction.

Digestive tract decreases peristalsis.

Secretion of digestive fluids decreases.

Adrenal glands stimulate adrenalin secretion, increasing blood sugar, blood pressure, and heart rate.

Secretions of the pancreas decrease.

Liver releases sugar into the bloodstream.

Urinary bladder relaxes.

Urinary sphincter closes.

Anal sphincter closes.

Blood vessels in external genitalia dilate.

How the body responds to stress . . . The Stress Response.

The stress response How the body responds internally is closely associated with Hans Selye's Stress Response (or General Adaptation Syndrome) Theory. His theory resulted from extensive research on animals and humans. Concluding that animals, including people, respond similarly when experiencing stress, Selye described three distinct phases of the stress response.

The first phase or stage is the *alarm reaction*, consisting of the automatic activation of the endocrine and sympathetic nervous systems. Under the danger of physical harm, for example, the brain perceives the danger, quickly activates the hypothalamus and pituitary glands and in turn stimulates the outpouring of hormones and nerve impulses. Nearly every vital function of the body is altered during the alarm reaction. The components of the alarm reaction, therefore, energizes our body for action—giving us a fast-responding and natural survival mechanism.

The second component of the Stress Response is the *resistance* (or adaptive) phase. During this phase the body attempts to repair and restore its internal state. The parasympathetic nervous system is more active, and the changes brought about by the alarm reaction are reversed. During this phase the body repairs any tissue damage and restores its adaptive energies, namely liver and muscle glycogen. In this manner the body is able to successfully manage subsequent episodes of stress manifested by the alarm reaction.

If stress continues unabated and the body is not given sufficient time to repair or restore itself, the adaptive energies, according to Selye, may be diminished. Selye calls this the stage of *exhaustion*. He believes that the so-called diseases of adaptation are likely to occur when the human organism reaches the exhaustion phase of the stress response. The cardiovascular system (heart disease), the renal system (kidney failure), the gastrointestinal system (ulcers), the endocrine system (hyperthyroidism) or the immune system (cancer) may suffer a breakdown in function.

Selye also contends that it is possible that the general storehouse of adaptive energies may become depleted, which could lead to early senility and shortened longevity.

Sounding the alarm Can you imagine the amount of anxiety and tension a cave dweller would have if we could suddenly place him behind the wheel of an automobile in a fast-paced metropolis like New York City? His basic instincts and techniques for survival might not hold up very well.

You and the cave dweller of more than 150,000 years ago have something in common: Your body and his react identically to stress. When faced with physical danger, your body, like his, prepares either to run or fight. What you have that the cave dweller did not is a highly complex technological society to survive in. You must survive the anxieties caused by worry, fears,and negative attitudes about hundreds of events that affect your life, but over which you have little or no control. Experts feel that the conflicts that exist between the biological you and the cultural you may lead to distress.

Today we perhaps face fewer direct real threats to our lives, but we have difficulty coping with the apparent or perceived threats we do face. We often become distressed over events which directly assault our self-esteem, our dignity, and our self-image. We worry about grades, our job, our money, our children, our appearance, our personal relationships, big government, big corporations, world hunger, world politics and global disaster.

The stress and health connection

One of the most insidious health problems over the last several decades has been our inability to resolve the biological-cultural conflict and deal with the tensions and stresses it has caused. Perhaps we were mistakenly looking for external causes of these stress-inflicted diseases. We perhaps made another error by looking for external miracle cures as well. Today the challenge is clear. We must manage stress within ourselves. We must look inside ourselves to resolve our stress conflicts. Many Americans have already done so. For them, a "wellness revolution" has begun.

Stressors

Insel and Roth define a stressor as "any demand giving rise to a coping response."[5] Some writers have categorized stressors as social, psychological, psycho-social, physical and philosophical. Others working in business and industry have identified stressors as organizational and environmental. Still others prefer no labels, but identify specific life events that act as stressors. These life events are generally listed according to the relative degree of stress they produce. They might range from a ticket for a minor traffic violation to the death of a close friend or family member.

It is important to recognize that most human activities are potential stressors. Conflicts with other persons, poor time management, ineffective communication, changes in jobs or geographical locations, illness and injuries, changes in economic or social status, crowding, confinement, marriage, divorce, sexual difficulties, conflict in value or belief systems and poor nutrition are examples of stressors that routinely exist in our daily lives.

Tolerance factors Do stressors affect people in exactly the same way? Why is it that at a time of crisis one person may become totally immobilized while another may remain calm and systematically take appropriate action?

Have you ever witnessed or participated in an event that created distress in one person but eustress in another? Most of us have. For example, some people are genuinely frightened by a roller-coaster ride, whereas others feel exhilarating joy. Some people laugh then they spill soda all over their new jeans, while other get angry. Some students show extreme anxiety and tension just before an exam, while others remain calm and collected. Each of us tolerates stress differently because we are unique, each having a different set of genetic material which may influence our behavior. A certain body structure, for example, may allow us to tolerate certain physical or environmental stresses better than others.

The entire range of socio-cultural experiences may determine how we tolerate psycho-social stressors. Perhaps being alone in the woods at night does not frighten you because you grew up on a farm. But you might feel very insecure (stressful) in a crowded city, as opposed to someone who grew up there. Your previous experiences and degree of practice or training in given events and situations can also influence how well you deal with them when you encounter them a second time.

It is difficult to predict how an individual will react to a *new* stressor. Each of us may differ somewhat in our ability to separate real threats from imaginary ones. Gradual and intensive training can help us deal more effectively with real stress and worry less about the imaginary kind.

At any given time in our lives, our philosophy of life may affect our tolerance for stress. Our basic value system and what we morally believe can support us at times of crisis. People who are spiritually strong and feel secure about their own existence and purpose in life seem to tolerate stress well.

The amount of social support we have is perhaps the most important factor in stress tolerance. Having a wide circle of friends or close family ties gives us a sense of importance and of belonging. When solid friends are there to lean on occasionally or to listen to our deepest concerns, we tend to move more easily through life's crises. A good social support system, which could take the form of a team, a club, an organization or a few close personal friends, is a definite asset for each of us.

THE SOCIAL SUPPORT SCALE

High Support = 70 or more   Moderate = 40 to 69   Low = less than 40

1. Do you belong to any of these kinds of groups? If YES, please indicate how much you take part in group activities. For example, VERY ACTIVE means you attend most meetings; SOMEWHAT ACTIVE means you attend meetings once in a while; INACTIVE means that you belong, but hardly ever go to meetings.

	DO YOU BELONG?	INACTIVE	SOMEWHAT ACTIVE	VERY ACTIVE
a. A social or recreational group?	1☐NO 2☐YES	1☐	2☐	3☐
b. A labor union, commercial group, or professional association?	1☐NO 2☐YES 1☐NO 2☐YES	1☐ 1☐	2☐ 2☐	3☐ 3☐
c. A political-party group or club?	1☐NO 2☐YES	1☐	2☐	3☐
d. A group concerned with children? (Such as P.T.A. or Boy Scouts)	1☐NO 2☐YES	1☐	2☐	3☐
e. A group concerned with community betterment, charity, or service?	1☐NO 2☐YES	1☐	2☐	3☐

ASIDE FROM THE ABOVE GROUPS,
DO YOU BELONG TO:

	DO YOU BELONG?	INACTIVE	SOMEWHAT ACTIVE	VERY ACTIVE
f. A church-connected group?	1☐NO 2☐YES	1☐	2☐	3☐
g. A group concerned with a public issue such as civil liberties, property rights, etc.?	1☐NO 2☐YES	1☐	2☐	3☐
h. A group concerned with the environment, pollution, etc.?	1☐NO 2☐YES	1☐	2☐	3☐
i. A group concerned with self-improvement that meets regularly?	1☐NO 2☐YES	1☐	2☐	3☐
j. Any other groups?	1☐NO 2☐YES	1☐	2☐	3☐

Describe them: _____

The score is found by adding all the numbers next to the box.

Overload signals The control of stress-causing tensions begin with the recognition of overload signs. These signals warn us that our adaptive energies may be low. They tell us of possible impending and serious episodes of distress. When mild, the signals may cause us to lose our vitality and sense of direction temporarily. As the signals intensify, a serious breech of our health and functioning capacity is likely to occur.

A partial list of overload signals gathered from Steinmetz[6] and others includes: headaches, general body weakness, dizziness, stomach aches, backaches, stiff neck or shoulders, pounding heart, nervous tics, impulsive behavior, inability to concentrate, forgetfulness, compulsive eating or non-eating, compulsive smoking, impatience, non-specific anxieties, increased use of drugs or alcohol, insomnia, depression, worrying, crying, blaming, frustration, loneliness, powerlessness and inflexibility.

We often begin to show signs of stress when our expectations are not met. Repeated disappointments sometimes lead to frustration, then feelings of helplessness and possibly to irrational acts. Although this is the exception rather than the rule, recall the story of the forty-one-year-old Jim Tyrer. Jim was a 6-foot 4-inch, 270-pound All-Pro offensive tackle for the Kansas City Chiefs. Following his retirement Jim tried at least four different business ventures. All of them failed and Jim fell into debt.

Jim Tyrer was one man who never gave up—he was not a quitter. He even moved into a smaller house to reduce the mortgage payments in order to keep his children in private schools. Jim's salary dropped from $80,000 a year as a player to $25,000. Overworking to maintain his financial status and his self-respect, Jim's adaptive energies eventually ran out. On a late-summer evening in 1980, in the bedroom of his home, Jim Tyrer shot and killed his wife and himself—a tragic story of too much stress.

Learn to recognize these subtle signs for what they are—signals telling us that our stress-handling capacities are being overloaded. Keep track of when they occur and associate them with events which may bring them about. You may also wish to examine your general personality type, as described by Friedman and Rosenman.[7]

Friedman and Rosenman contend that there is a direct relationship between a certain personality type and heart disease. According to their studies, Type-A persons exhibit "hurry sickness," "time urgency," and other impatient behaviors. The opposite Type-B, person is more relaxed and deliberate in his personal and work behaviors.

Remember, the first step toward effectively controlling your daily stress is recognition of the overstress signals.

Controlling Stress

All of us desire to feel that we are in control of ourselves. We like to feel in command of our own behaviors and readily able to manage our daily personal and occupational tasks. We feel good about ourselves when we sense a purpose and a direction to our lives.

All of us face frequent and daily episodes of stress. We sometimes control the stress level through muscle tension-releasing methods or through meditation (looking inward). Often we control stress by seeking a diversion or a change of pace to recharge our draining batteries. In a real sense, each of us possesses our own stress-control mechanisms. These controls are the powers which lie within each of us.

The Relaxation Response[8]

A focal point of many of the stress-control and tension-reduction methods is what Benson defines as the Relaxation Response. According to Benson, it is the physiological opposite of Selye's Stress Response. In the Stress Response our internal mechanisms are "geared up." In the Relaxation Response, they are "geared down."

Benson contends that the relaxation response is as *natural* as the stress response and that in the modern era we are just beginning to relearn how to elicit its beneficial effects.

STRESS CONTROL METHODS

Effective coping One of the foremost authorities in developing techniques to help people reduce tension (often undetectable muscle contractions) is Edmund Jacobsen, M.D.[9] In his Chicago Laboratory for Clinical Physiology, Dr. Jacobsen did extensive research on the subject of stress and tension control. It was here that he developed his famous Progressive Relaxation techniques.

Jacobsen, with his extensive work in the field, pioneered the use of electrophysiological apparatus to study stress reduction.

In fact, many of the more sophisticated biofeedback systems used widely today were born in Jacobsen's laboratory.

Most stress control techniques, methods and guidelines essentially come to one common point: The individual must consciously release body (muscular) tensions. The individual must have a sincere desire to make a behavioral change and must be willing to devote effort to train for a permanent change.

To be effective, the coping strategy should be appropriate to the individual, but professional assistance by trained specialists is available if the person wishes it. As a precaution, however, medical consultation is warranted and recommended as a first step when signs or symptoms of illness or disease are present.

The following is a partial listing of some of the more general methods which may be useful in tension control and stress management:

Progressive relaxation is a program whereby the person is taught to recognize and eliminate excessive muscle tension. Following recognition of tension, the individual is trained to tense, then consciously relax the various skeletal muscles. The person may have to perform the actions several times daily until they become habitual. Muscle groups are usually relaxed in sequence, progressing from the feet up through the body to the face and head. An excellent resource on relaxation techniques was written by Curtis and Detert.[10]

Biofeedback is an electronic means to self-monitor physiological states, particularly the small muscle contractions existing deep in muscle tissue. Through electronic sound or image, the person hears or sees his own muscle tensions, which enables him to become aware of the causes of the tension. The system is painless, with small electrodes leading from the practitioner's forehead into the biofeedback instrument. The technique is designed to help the person reach a deeper awareness of the feelings, thoughts or emotions that may lie at the root of stress. As a diagnostic or training device, biofeedback is an excellent tool to promote self-exploration, self-awareness and self-control.

Meditation and body awareness programs are primarily designed to bring the practitioner peace of mind and to enhance positive thinking. Tension control and stress management are often by-products of the process. A wide range of methodology, some within a religious context and some not, has been invented.

As a 1976 *Newsweek* writer put it, there are 8,000 ways to "awaken" in North America. Some of the better-known autogenic programs include TM (Transcendental Meditation), EST, ARICA, Silva Mind Control, Rolfing, Feldenkrais Training, Psychosynthesis, Guided Fantasy and Bioenergetics. Before embarking on such programs, it is suggested that you discuss them with professionals who are familiar with their advantages and disadvantages.

Regular exercise can be one of the most effective stress control devices available. Nearly everyone can exercise, but it should be regular, ego-void and non-competitive to be most effective. Aerobic exercises (walking, dancing, jogging, running, swimming, cycling) burn up the powerful energy created by stress and leave the body and mind quietly relaxed.

A highly competitive once- or twice-a-week racquetball game or tennis match may be adding stress to your fast-paced life rather than reducing it. Exercises such as yoga (although not usually considered an aerobically-stimulating activity), does promote deep relaxation and stress reduction. In addition to physical exertion, many exercise and sports programs provide diversion and refreshing changes of pace from our daily routine, and this also helps control stress.

Practical suggestions about controlling work stress and stress in general are numerous. Here are a few of them:

- Manage time effectively. Set priorities and do only what is reasonable and realistic.
- Negotiate realistic deadlines and avoid setting ones you know you cannot keep.
- Improve communications skills. Faulty communication is often a source of stress.
- Build support relationships by making new friends.
- Try to reduce the amount of daily trivia you must deal with.
- Eliminate work area noise and confusion if possible.
- When you have a break, take it. Don't get in the habit of working through breaks.
- Throughout the day, take an occasional five-minute break to relax and think.
- Plan ahead. Try to eliminate future stressors before they occur.
- Try to reduce polyphasic behavior. Concentrate on one task at a time.

- Do not let work dominate your life.
- Take action to settle problems as soon as possible. Do not let stress drift on and on.
- Guard your personal freedom and your private moments.
- Try new experiences, diversions and changes of pace.
- Practice making positive self-statements.
- Put more humor into your life.
- Spend some time outdoors daily.
- Maintain a comfortable and healthy level of body weight.
- Practice good nutrition habits and minimize the consumption of "junk" foods.
- Maintain regular and adequate sleep habits.

Ineffective coping Faulty or ineffective coping behaviors sometimes appear to bring temporary relief from stress, but in the long term they usually increase it. Poor coping methods can lead to serious illness and even death.

The more injurious and non-productive coping behaviors involve the use of artificial substances, such as narcotic drugs, patent drugs, over-prescribed prescription drugs or alcohol to relieve stress symptoms. In addition, compulsive smoking, eating or non-eating, caffeine ingestion and mega-vitamin or mega-nutrient intake may contribute to your stress. Any self-medication of substances which adversely change your physiology should be cleared by your physician. Individuals who are now using ineffective or dangerous coping behaviors to relieve stress should seek professional advice.

Some individuals attempt to control stress by avoiding it. Avoiding serious threats to your health or body through injury is prudent on your part. However, attempting to avoid *all* stress at all costs can prove to be stressful. This avoidance behavior generally promotes more stress because it is not a realistic expectation—in fact, it is nearly impossible. Remember, stress is basically a natural, constructive and *desirable* force in our lives. Realistically, you should strive to control, manage and use it to enhance the quality of your life.

MIDSHIPMEN AND STRESS

The daily demands upon the midshipmen at the U.S. Naval Academy are enormous. Daily schedules are filled with military, physical and academic training with time only for eating, studying and sleeping in preparation for more of the same the succeeding day. Except for brief holidays, leaves and social occasions the intense training of a Naval officer is unabated for four years.

How do the midshipmen manage these pressures (stressors)? What conditions prevail at the Academy and what personal behaviors enable the midshipmen to successfully handle this stress as it occurs daily? Let us examine some of the factors.

Realistic expectations The Naval Academy has established clear purposes for the training of U.S. Naval and Marine officers. For the fourth classmen—plebes—the pressures of Academy life begin each summer prior to the opening of the academic year in the fall. According to the catalogue, the aim of plebe training is to:

> Exercise self-discipline
> Organize time and effort effectively
> *Perform efficiently under stress*
> Think and react quickly with good judgement
> Exhibit an exemplary military bearing and appearance.

The Academy program is intentionally demanding. The candidates for admission must successfully pass rigorous medical, academic and physical standards for admission.

However, despite these standards each midshipmen usually finds one or more of the requirements severely challenging. As high achievers, the candidates on the whole are highly motivated toward success. Their attitude toward the rigor of the training is realistically within their potential. Stress often occurs when our expectations are set unrealistically too high for our abilities. Unmet expectations lead to frustration which may lead to stress.

Sense of belonging (social support) One of the most effective ways to deal with stress is to have a strong social support group which respects and appreciates your efforts and which can share your joys and your disappointments.

As a military training institution, the Naval Academy assigns each fourth class midshipman to a military unit and subunit. Generally, the midshipmen remain attached to the same units throughout their four years. Various competitive and non-competitive activities which foster leadership, teamwork and cooperation are organized and carried out regularly. These groups often serve as effective surrogate family and identity groups, just as those that exist in regular civilian life for young people.

Established controls and self-discipline The Naval Academy's regulations regarding personal actions and behavior are clearly spelled out and understood by the midshipmen. Essentially, there is no confusion in the midshipmen's mind about proper conduct, about who is in control, and about what the consequences of misconduct are.

Stress in our work and personal lives sometimes results when we do not clearly understand our roles and the roles of those with whom we interact daily. Although roles do change, there should be effective communication indicating that this has happened.

Exercise and fitness The Naval Academy provides—in fact requires—a rigorous program of exercise and sports participation by all midshipmen. When performed regularly and properly, exercise and sports improve one's tolerance against physical and psychological stress. It also provides a positive and beneficial outlet for the release of stress-accumulated energies.

Stress tends to accumulate in individuals who do not have effective control techniques or who are unable to physically release this abundant energy from time to time.

Nutrition and adequate rest
The Naval Academy provides a highly nutritious and balanced diet for the midshipmen. Although the amount of food eaten is a personal matter and can lead to weight problems, the meals are regular and well-prepared. Some experts believe that a poor diet can bring about stress. Since plebes are required to eat breakfast, good habits of eating are established early in the midshipman's training. One of the keys to good nutrition is to eat a variety of foods to achieve an adequate balance of all essential nutrients, including carbohydrates, fats, proteins, vitamins and minerals.

Providing adequate rest for the body is another hedge against accumulated stress. Cutting in on important and regular sleep habits is not recommended. Although the amount of sleep required varies from individual to individual, the general recommendation is between seven and eight hours a night if afternoon naps are not taken. At the USNA taps are at 11:00 P.M. and reveille at 6:00 A.M.

Social and recreational outlets Having social, recreational and personal diversions from the heavy load of routine work is healthy and helps control stress. The Naval Academy provides opportunities for such activities. Attendance at athletic events, social events and cultural programs is encouraged. One of the early signs of stress exists when one refuses to participate in any type of outlet activities. In addition, resources such as the use of a quiet chapel for introspection, attendance at religious services or informal meetings with officers and faculty are useful stress deterrents.

Recognition for personal effort
Some of the most stressful occupations in typical American life are those where personal effort is not recognized or rewarded. Midshipmen on the whole clearly see the results of their efforts. In the short term the accomplishment of each course and each special type of training brings the midshipman closer to a long-range goal. They recognize that their efforts will eventually pay off as a highly recognized and respected U.S. naval officer.

The thought that the difficult training will enable one to serve and defend the United States brings a sense of pride and elation to a young career officer. When such dreams and expectations are kept close to reality, a sense of inner security and confidence is achieved.

Whether you are a midshipman, a college or high school student, a retired executive or a home caregiver, stress must be handled on a very personal basis. Those who take stress as it comes, prepare themselves physically and psychologically for it and approach life with a positive and enthusiastic spirit will adjust exceedingly well. Even the major crises that we all must face periodically can be handled effectively. The ability to manage stress is an important component of your personal health and fitness program throughout your life.

The advice which Heinz Lenz gives his midshipmen about stress is:

The idea is not to eliminate the butterflies, but to get them to fly in formation.

REFERENCES

1. Selye, Hans. *The Stress of Life* (Rev. ed.). New York: McGraw-Hill, 1976.
2. Girdano, Daniel A. and George S. Everly, *Controlling Stress and Tension: A Holistic Approach.* Englewood Cliffs: Prentice-Hall, 1979, p. 5.
3. Brown, Barbara B., *Super-Mind: The Ultimate Energy.* New York: Harper and Row, 1980, p. 90.
4. Toffler, Alvin, *Future Shock.* New York: Random House, 1970.
5. Insel, Paul M. and Walton T. Roth, *Core Concepts in Health.* Palo Alto: Mayfield Publishing Co., 3rd Ed., p. 19.
6. Steinmetz, Jenny et al., *Managing Stress.* Palo Alto: Bull Publishing Co., 1980, p. 5.
7. Friedman, Meyer and Ray H. Rosenman, *Type A Behavior and Your Heart.* Greenwich, Connecticut: Fawcett Publications, 1974.
8. Benson, Herbert, *The Relaxation Response.* New York: Wm. Morrow and Co. 1975.
9. Jacobsen, Edmund, *You Must Relax.* New York: McGraw-Hill, 1962.
10. Curtis, John D. and Richard A. Detert. *How to Relax: A Holistic Approach to Stress Management.* Palo Alto: Mayfield Publishing Co., 1981.

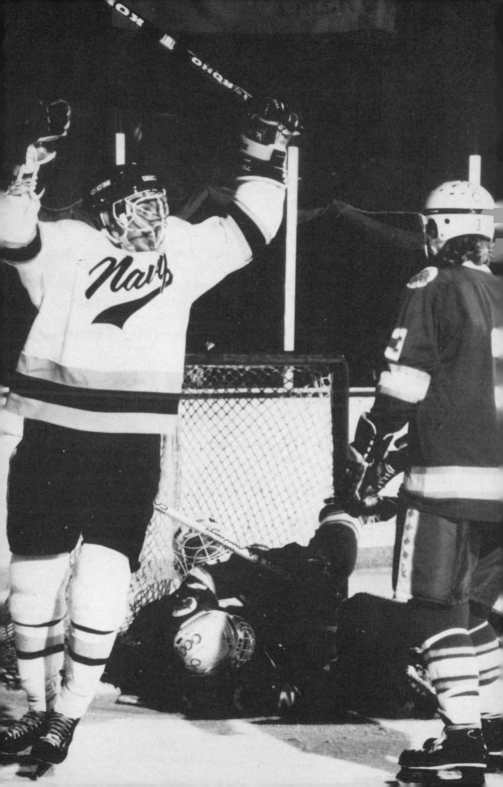

10

EXERCISE AND FITNESS INJURIES

The grueling race begins at 7 A.M. from the Kailua-Kona Pier on Hawaii's largest island of Hawaii with a 2.4-mile ocean swim, followed by a 112-mile bike race and a 26.2-mile marathon.

Description of
the Ironman Triathlon
USA Today, October 8, 1982

OBJECTIVES

- Identify some of the probable signals associated with oncoming exercise injuries.
- List the most common types of exercise injuries.
- Describe the general causes of exercise injuries.
- Explain how exercise injuries can be prevented or minimized.
- Examine the usual methods and procedures in the treatment and rehabilitation of exercise injuries.

Another fitness-related health factor which the exerciser should consider is the possible injuries that may occur during favorite sport or fitness activities.

The risk of physical injury is the athlete's nemesis. Nearly all who decide that exercise, fitness and athletic participation is an important part of their lives will likely experience some physical discomfort, soreness or injury at some time. This is inevitable, and for many it is an acceptable risk of participation. However, by conditioning properly, taking certain precautions and staying well within one's limitations, there is an excellent chance that injuries from participation can be prevented or minimized.

In this chapter attention will focus on the more general considerations regarding exercise and fitness injuries. The underlying theme, however, will be that the prevention of activity-restricting and debilitating injuries is far more prudent than attempting to correct the problem once it has developed.

Because the prevention of injuries should be a major priority for the exerciser, as well as for the competitive athlete, the advice offered by Robert Buxbaum[1] appears sound. Buxbaum states that there are four points to keep in mind when attempting to prevent or lessen the severity of sports injuries. They are:

- Match the sport to the individual. For example, a person who is excessively obese and suffers from knee injuries should not start out on a jogging program. Perhaps a walking or swimming starter program would be more appropriate.
- Train specifically and condition yourself for the sport. This pre-participation conditioning program should include specific muscular strength, endurance, flexibility and cardiovascular exercises required by the sport.
- Modify the rules of the sport, if necessary. Not all sports have to be played by the rules of the book. Modify them and the playing conditions (with prior agreement by all participants, of course) when the chance of personal injuries can be lessened.
- Use appropriate protective equipment. If participation in the sport is known to cause certain types of injuries, then by all means protect yourself, regardless of how ridiculous or less macho it may appear to others.

EARLY WARNING SIGNALS

There are early warning signs that an exerciser or athlete should not ignore. They may indicate that your current workout schedule or program is causing a physiological or anatomical change which may lead to a more serious injury or disturbance.

Sheehan[2] states that when the athlete is at his peak, he is just a hair's breadth away from being overtrained. Elaborating somewhat on some of the warning signs identified in Sheehan's *The Encyclopedia of Athletic Medicine*, the following represent signals which even the novice exerciser can interpret to mean that an injury may be pending unless one slows down:

- **Decline in performance.** There are both physical and psychological causes of this, perhaps the first indication that the body needs a rest. A decline in performance, for whatever reason, is telling you that you may be overworking your body.
- **Loss of weight.** Another possible signal of impending physical problems for the athlete is weight loss that occurs without conscious effort to reduce caloric intake or lose weight.
- **Elevated resting pulse rate.** George Sheehan relies on his resting pulse rate as a barometer of readiness to perform additional work. When the pulse rate is well above normal rate Sheehan does not work out that day.
- **Labored breathing.** When breathing becomes a chore, especially during aerobic activities which normally are performed with easy breathing, this may be an early sign of body fatigue.
- **Sleeplessness.** The inability to sleep soundly may be a result of overly stiff muscles, pain from muscle or joint injuries or a disturbance of metabolic activity. Sleeplessness often results from some type of stress which may be caused by overworking or overexercising.
- **Changes in bowel or bladder patterns.** Noticeable changes in your usual bowel or bladder habits may occur during the early onset of fatigue. The fatigue could likely result from improper or too much training.

- **Pain.** Muscle and joint pain is a sure sign that your body may not be responding well to your type of training or skill movements. Pain should never be ignored because it is your body's way of signalling you that something is wrong. Do not try to "run through" severe pain.
- **Fatigue.** Exercise should help promote an energetic lifestyle, not deprive you of it. Fatigue may also be an important early warning signal.

   Fatigue is an interesting and complex phenomenon. Researchers have demonstrated the effects of fatiguing local muscle groups. However, general fatigue is more complex and less well understood its causes may be psychological, physiological or a combination of both. A change of pace, routine or activity often relieves general feelings of fatigue.
- **Appetite.** Diminished or excessive appetite may be signals of too severe an exercise program.
- **Thirst.** Excessive thirst long after cessation of your workout may also indicate some disturbance of your internal physiology. It is wise to monitor thirst.
- **Psychological changes.** The "blahs"—lack of enthusiasm, lack of confidence and just general "staleness" feelings—often infect regular exercisers and athletes. By recognizing these signs one can easily shift to a new routine to provide a diversion from regular, humdrum training. Often a short (and guilt-free) vacation from physical effort is needed to regenerate your enthusiasm for the activity once again.

COMMON EXERCISE INJURIES

The scope of this text permits only a very general discussion of exercise injuries. The reader is directed to other excellent and comprehensive athletic injuries texts if greater detail and depth of understanding is desired.

Fahey, in his simply written and easy-to-understand book *What to do About Athletic Injuries,*[3] defines four broad categories of injuries. These include 1) sudden traumatic injuries (blows to the head, sharp blows which break bones, and so on); 2) repeated traumatic injuries (as with a boxer being repeatedly struck on the head); 3) overuse injuries (tennis elbow and achilles tendonitis);

and 4) imbalance injuries (over or underdeveloped antagonistic muscle groups, or anatomical weaknesses).

Unless a regular exerciser is competing in a contact sport or a sport involving the control over a special piece of equipment (for example a bicycle), most exercise and fitness injuries arise from overuse or muscle imbalance. Overuse simply means that you have overextended your capacity to perform a given activity at your present level of condition. Imbalance injuries generally result when certain activities favor training of muscle groups over their antagonistic opposite muscle group. In certain instances, because of surgery, disease, disorder or heredity, certain muscle groups are too weak to perform in balance with other muscle groups. These would also be classified as muscle imbalance injuries.

It should be remembered that for the most part many exercise and fitness injuries are caused by muscle imbalance and overuse. Most of these injuries also involve the tissue closely surrounding the joints, particularly the lower extremities. Sheehan[4] indicates that the three leading injuries affecting runners include knee injuries (17.9%), Achilles tendon problems (14.0%) and shin splints (10.6%). Injuries to the major leg muscles are somewhat less frequent: calves (3.6%), hamstrings (2.6%) and thighs (1.3%).

If most of your exercise is obtained through participation in individual sports like tennis or racquetball, or through team sports like basketball or soccer, sudden traumatic and repeated traumatic injuries to other parts of the body are more likely. Many of the most common injuries sustained are included in the following brief (and noninclusive) list, regardless of the sport or exercise activity:

COMMON EXERCISE INJURIES

- **Abrasion:** A friction injury causing damage to the outer layer of skin.

- **Blister:** An injury caused by friction which results in a bubble beneath the skin.

- **Bruise:** A "black-and-blue" injury caused by blood leaking into the damaged tissue.

- **Bursitis:** Inflammation of any of the bursa, sac-like structures in joints—especially ball-and-socket joints.

- **Cramp:** A painful muscle spasm, often in the gastrocnemius (calf) muscle.

- **Dehydration:** A serious condition for the exerciser, caused by a loss or insufficient supply of water in the body.

- **Frostbite:** A possible cold weather injury in which exposed skin is frozen.

- **Heat Exhaustion:** A condition where the individual perspires profusely and is weak with possible dizziness. The skin is pale and clammy, and the body temperature close to normal.

- **Heat stroke:** A serious condition where the body temperature is dangerously high and skin is hot, red and dry. The sweating mechanism has been blocked.

- **Shin splint:** A painful injury involving the anterior portion of the lower leg.

- **Sprain:** An injury involving damage to a ligament or joint capsule.

- **Strain:** A common injury which overstretches a muscle or its tendon.

- **Spasm:** A forceful involuntary contraction of a specific muscle or muscle group.

- **Stress Fracture:** An injury resulting in damage directly to a bone.

- **Tendonitis:** Inflammation of a tendon, usually as a result of repeated use and stress.

Exercisers should also be alert to the more serious disorders which may be experienced during or following activity. These would include respiratory and cardiac-related dysfunctions. In these instances exercise should be terminated immediately and a physician consulted.

PREVENTING AND MINIMIZING INJURIES

Besides Buxbaum's advice at the beginning of this chapter, there are other considerations which may help prevent or minimize sports and exercise injuries.

Perhaps the main factor to keep in mind during your conditioning program is not to overtrain. If you prefer to work out five to seven times a week, follow a hard-easy schedule. Be sure to avoid ultra-strict schedules which might cause you to work out at times when you are injured or when rest from fatigue will be more valuable to your training. Also maintain a good diet and use quality equipment, especially well-constructed shoes.

The following injury preventive suggestions will also help if you adhere to them. View them as the do's and don't's of injury prevention.

- Do condition yourself very gradually to avoid overuse injuries.

- Do condition your body at least several weeks prior to participating in a *competitive* sports program.

- Do acclimatize your body or reduce exertion if you exercise at high altitudes.

- Do take adequate amounts of nutrients and fluids to sustain your exercise intensity or coincide with environmental factors such as heat and humidity.

- Do use flexibility exercises regularly, especially before and after strenuous exercise workouts. (Poor flexibility is an important cause of exercise and fitness injuries.)

- Do not initiate a vigorous (competitive) exercise program without a thorough medical and physical evaluation.

- Do not exercise in hot/humid weather unless you have gradually acclimatized yourself properly. (See guidelines in the Appendix.)

- Do not exercise when the air quality is at poor or dangerous levels, especially if you have respiratory or circulatory system disorders.

- Do not exercise on terrain or surfaces that increase your risk of injury. When competing in a sports contest where injuries are possible, be certain that medical assistance is readily available.

- Do not exercise when you are seriously ill with infections or other disorders that may further endanger your health. When experiencing unusual or severe *pain*, stop exercising immediately.

- Do not use drugs or special nutrients to enhance performance without appropriate and prior medical consultation.

TREATING EXERCISE INJURIES

As participation in fitness and sports activities continues to increase at the current phenomenal rate, more specialists will be trained in various branches of the rapidly growing science of sports medicine. Because the medical community has now accepted sports medicine as a specialty, better diagnostic treatment and rehabilitative programs and techniques are likely to emerge. These trends will certainly benefit everyone who decides that keeping fit is a lifetime experience that will lead to a higher quality of life.

But what should the average person know about the treatment of injuries? First, it is important to know that excellent injury treatment centers do exist throughout the country. Most cities in the United States with professional athletic teams have excellent sports medicine centers with trained staffs. Most of these centers accept professional as well as non-professional athletes for treatment. Second, there are excellent books currently available which provide sound advice about preventing injuries, what to do if you are injured, and how to care for minor athletic injuries. You may wish to check the references at the end of this chapter. Third, you can follow the briefly outlined advice given in the following section if you do sustain an exercise or sport injury.

WHAT TO DO WHEN AN INJURY OCCURS

Southmayd and Hoffman,[5] excerpting from Mirkin's excellent text, recommend the *RICE* procedure for most exercise or athletic injuries. The formula means: Rest (continuing the exercise may further extend the injury), Ice (cold in the form of ice decreases bleeding from injured blood vessels), Compression (pressure usually from one type of wrapping limits swelling) and Elevation (keeping the injured part above the heart helps drain excess fluid). The procedure should be used for up to 24 hours, and caution should be taken that the compression wrap does not cut off circulation.

Although not all minor injuries require examination by a physician, many injuries should be checked out to be certain that long-term damage is held to a minimum. Southmayd and Hoffman[6] (again excerpting from Mirkin) state that you should see a doctor when:

- The injury causes severe pain.
- The injury involves a joint or ligament.
- You cannot move the body part.
- There is pain in a joint or bone for more than two weeks.
- An injury does not heal in three weeks.
- An injury causes an infection (characterized by pus, red streaks, swollen lymph nodes or fever).

PREVENTION IS THE BEST MEDICINE

By following some of the general suggestions presented in this unit, you may be practicing the best medicine of all—prevention. To remain injury-free in order to obtain the pleasures and joy of physical activity should be a goal for every exerciser and fitness-conscious person.

REFERENCES

1. Buxbaum, Robert, *Sports for Life*. Boston: Beacon Press, 1979, pp. 62-63.
2. Sheehan, George A., *The Encyclopedia of Athletic Medicine*. Mountain View, CA.: World Publications, 1972, pp. 14-15.
3. Fahey, Thomas D., *What to do About Athletic Injuries (How to Prevent, How to Treat Them)*. New York: Butterick Publishing, 1979, p.33.

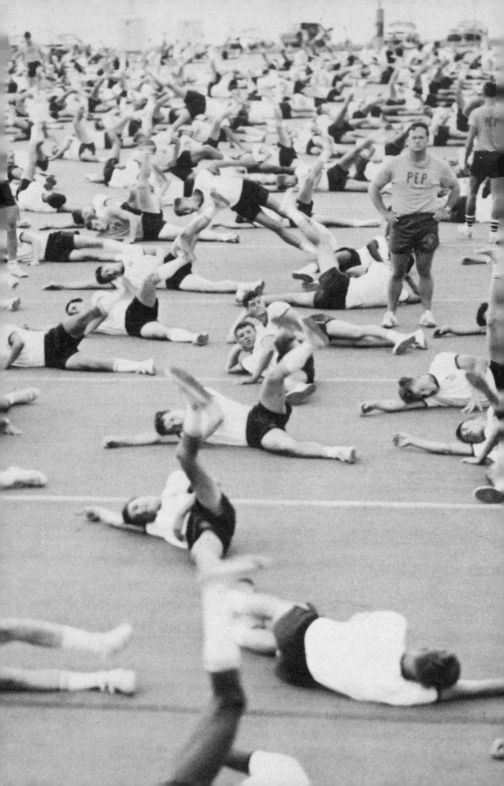

4. Sheehan, George A., op. cit., p. 24.
5. Southmayd, William and Marshall Hoffman, *Sports Health: The Complete Book of Athletic Injuries.* New York: Quick Fox Press, 1981, pp. 40-41.
6. ibid., pp. 41-42.

Additional sources

Appenzeller, Otto and Ruth A. Atkinson, *Sports Medicine: Fitness, Training, Injuries.* Baltimore: Urban & Schwarzenberg, 1983, second edition.

Mirkin, Gabe, *The Sportsmedicine Book.* Boston: Little-Brown, 1978.

McGregor, Rob Roy and Stephen E. Devereaux, *EEVeTeC.* *Boston: Houghton Mifflin Company, 1982.*

Roy, Steven and Richard Irvin, Sports Medicine: Prevention, Evaluation, Management, and Rehabilitation. Englewood Cliffs: Prentice-Hall, 1983.

Sheehan, George A., *Medical Advice for Runners.* Mountain View, CA.: World Publications, 1978.

Strauss, Richard H., *Sports Medicine and Physiology.* Philadelphia: W.B. Saunders Company, 1979.

◄A flexible athlete is less prone to injury.

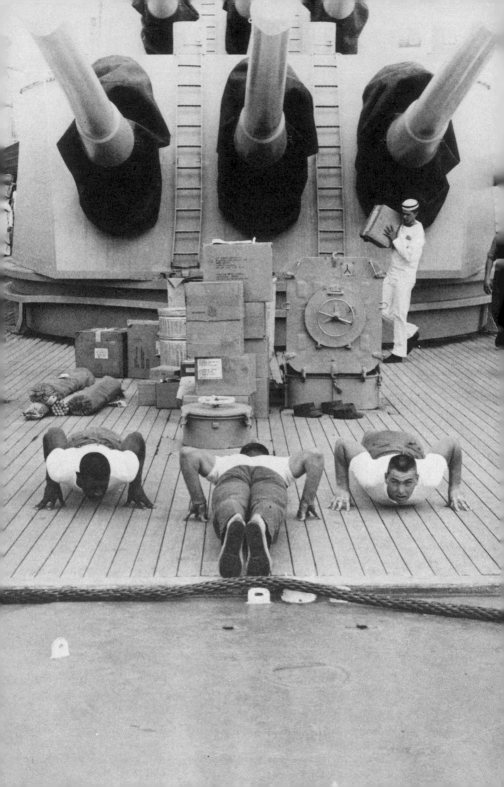

11

FITNESS ABOARD SHIP FOR SAILORS, AVIATORS AND MARINES

Mens Sana in Corpore sano

—D. Junius Juvenalis, 110 B.C.

OBJECTIVES

- Review the importance of mental alertness and physical readiness aboard ship.
- Discuss the role physical fitness has played in the Navy throughout the recent decades.
- Describe a practical evaluation of physical fitness aboard ship.
- Discuss possible facilities and activities on various ships of the fleet.
- Describe advanced training and testing programs underway.
- Point out the desirability of training while underway (at sea).

IMPORTANCE OF FITNESS READINESS ABOARD SHIP

It is interesting to see that in 110 B.C. a scholarly man, D.J. Juvenalis, declared that it was important to have a healthy mind in a healthy body. In fact, throughout the ages few men have denied the importance of developing not only the intellectual being, but the physical as well. Whether deployment and sea duty are scheduled for six months or a lengthy tour of 24 months, the Navy has always recognized that fighting the sea, the elements and wartime enemies from a fragile, seagoing platform requires well-trained, determined and physically fit men.

Going to sea has changed: ships have become sturdier, and the Navy's emphasis is more on the sailor's technological training than his physical capabilities. The fleet needs men who are trained in nuclear power, electronics and surface warfare skills. The superbly conditioned sailor can be of no assistance unless he is qualified in professional and technological areas as well. There is no question about it—this shift of emphasis has a bearing on the level of physical fitness of the seagoing men.

Yet the need for a high level of physical fitness cannot be ignored. It is the human being that keeps the technology aboard ship effective. It is the human being who carries out the skills of surface warfare.

It is a documented fact. The human being can be no more effective, regardless of preparation and skills, than his level of energy, well-being and physical fitness. Let us turn to a specific example.

One of the most exciting aspects of going to sea is to be involved in flight operations of an aircraft carrier. However, a great deal of danger is involved. It is of interest to note that accidents occur at a far greater rate after long hours of operation when personnel are fatigued. It might be argued that accidents are caused by factors other than the human being, but research has shown that it is the personnel that causes accidents. Table 1 supports this statement.

The author of the article from which the graphs shown in Table I are taken is Admiral E.S. McGinley II, USN (ret.).[1] The admiral states that there is "an inescapable tie-in with our system safety analyses: Almost every 'event' deduced is directly or indirectly related to human judgments, reactions or physical capabilities."

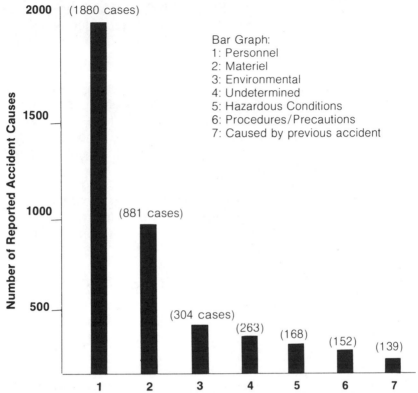

Table 1. Causes of Naval Ship Accidents, Fiscal Years 1970-1972

The Navy has long recognized that a high degree of physical fitness delays the onset of those conditions causing accidents and has for decades asserted the importance of physical fitness. The following is a brief historical review of physical fitness in the Navy.

Historical review

Prior to 1961 there had been no consistent Navy policy of fitness, which was considered the responsibility of the individual. On July 18, 1961, with the physical fitness awareness created by President Kennedy as its impetus, the Department of Defense issued a memorandum on the subject. It established physical fitness as an element of combat readiness and established required physical conditioning for all military personnel below 40 years of age. The instructions were contained in document number 6100.2 published by the Bureau of Personnel.

This document, BUPERSINST 6100.2, established standards and set up testing requirements throughout the Navy, but unfortunately it has not been totally effective.

Every ship in the Navy is periodically evaluated in two areas— according to its administrative operations and its combat readiness. Despite the emphasis of the instruction, the physical fitness requirements fell into the administrative domain rather than combat readiness, and thus physical fitness would be considered only as important as the commanding officer, the captain of the ship, chose to make it. Since captains are a product of the society within which they live, in a majority of cases physical fitness was considered relatively unimportant. Still, the Navy has tried consistently and conscientiously to improve the level of physical fitness through the implementation of BUPERSINST 6100.2. The most recent development in its campaign is outlined below.

**The Navy's present fitness program—
OPNAV INSTRUCTION 6110.1B, October 1982**
After considerable research and preparation, the Navy has issued a new document, OPNAV Instruction 6110.1B. It places emphasis in the following areas:

- The weight requirement is based on the percentage of body fat content and not solely on height and weight limits.
- Programs are provided to improve nutritional habits and lifestyles for those who so desire.
- Guidance is provided to promote vigorous and active fitness activities.

The document contains physical readiness classification tables and test requirements, a description of test items, a height-weight screening table and percent-fat prediction tables for men and women. All Naval personnel, except those excused for medical reasons, must become fit and maintain a condition of health and physical readiness consistent with their duties. It is indicated that personnel should exercise three times a week for at least 30 minutes to stay fit. Commanding officers are to reward those who do.

The Navy has added one step that has long been overdue, that those who do not maintain the required health and physical fitness standards will have that noted in officer fitness reports and enlisted evaluations. In addition, those who fall below prescribed standards in physical fitness and body fat will be put into remedial training programs and may be considered for separation from the service if improvements are not recorded.

The stage is set. Not only does this document serve as a motivating force, but in today's society the climate is right to train for physical fitness. For the first time in the Navy, the commanding officers will become positively and productively involved. Thus, today's seafaring personnel have every opportunity to become fit, not only ashore, but at sea.

OPPORTUNITIES FOR FITNESS AT SEA

From the questions and concerns voiced to the authors, it is evident that there is a great deal of interest in being physically fit aboard ship and it became apparent that it would be a good idea to prepare a physical fitness guide for seagoing personnel. Sailors would be able to carry out this program under all conditions, in the smallest spaces. Such a program is described below.

A sailor's practical ship-board physical fitness program

First of all, you need to determine your present level of physical fitness. Have a friend test you on the items below. Once you know your relative status, you will know how to pace yourself. Work through the training routine (you might try the torpedo deck if there is one aboard your ship). Have your friend bring a wristwatch with a sweep second hand so that he can time you during the exercises.

After you have trained for a period of six weeks, you will have established an adequate foundation of physical fitness. You may wish to continue to train in the indicated manner, or you may wish to choose other methods of training described in this chapter.

Fitness facilities aboard ship

Aircraft carriers, battleships and cruisers Maintaining and improving physical fitness is a relatively simple task on a large ship, where training space is available.

Test Items	Points
1. PULL-UPS—Palms forward, full hang, pull chin over bar.	
8 or more, score	5
4 or more, score	3
3 or less, score	1

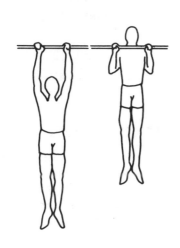

Test Items	Points
2. SIT-UPS (within 30 seconds)—Lie on back, arms over head, feet drawn up tight.	
25 sit-ups	5
18 sit-ups	3
10 sit-ups	1

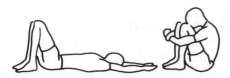

Test Items	Points
3. SIDE-STRADDLE HOP (60 seconds)—Your feet come apart as far as your shoulders are wide; arms swing up straight over shoulders.	
70 hops	5
60 hops	3
50 hops	1

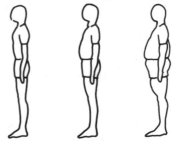

4. YOUR FIGURE.

If you look like (a), score	5
If you look like (b), score	3
If you look like (c), score	1

5. THE AGE FACTOR.

From 17 to 26 years old, score	0
From 27 to 38 years old, score	2
From 39 up, score	4

Now, add your total points. If they amount to 18 or more, consider your physical fitness status to be "excellent." Work in Group 1, described below.

If they range between 11 to 17, your condition is "Good." Work in Group II.

If they are 10 or less, that's too bad. You belong in the executive, or Group III, category.

At this point you are almost ready to begin to train. But first a few additional points should be observed.

1. Train in a space that is adequate and safe.
2. Adjust the repetitions to your own need, especially during the first weeks.
3. Train at least four out of seven days. Keep track on a calendar.
6. Observe carefully the principles outlined in the chapter on nutrition.
7. Weigh about once a week. Weigh on the same scales, at the same time, with the same amount of clothes each time. If you start your weighing before you work out do it that way every time. If after the workout, keep it that way. The point is, do it the same way each time. Keep track of your weight.
8. Now, let's look at your training routine. Program #1.

PROGRAM #1
GETTING IN SHAPE ABOARD SHIP

NOTE: REPS—This means "repetitions"; it means the number of times you repeat each exercise

SPD—This means the "speed" with which you do each exercise; there are three speeds

(1) SLOW—Move easily and work in relaxed manner

(2) MEDIUM—Move at a pace which is half as fast as you can go, abbreviated, "med"

(3) FAST—Move as fast as you can, still doing the exercise correctly

EXERCISE	PURPOSE	GROUP 3		GROUP 2		GROUP 1	
		REPS	SPD	REPS	SPD	REPS	SPD
STRETCHER—Feet apart shoulder width, arms over head, bend, and bounce, reaching for toes	Warm-up and for flexibility	15 to rt 13 to lt	slow	20 to rt 20 to lt	slow	20 to rt 20 to lt	slow
LOWER BACK EXERCISE—on head, feet drawn up to buttocks, heels touching buttocks.	Strength for lower back muscles	15	med.	20	med.	max you can do in 30 sec	fast
SIT-UPS—lie on back, arms over head, feet drawn up to buttocks heels touching buttocks	strength gut, good for stomach	17	med.	23	med.	max you can do in 30 sec	fast
TRUNK MUSCLES—lie on right side use right arm as brace, lift right leg high, lower, don't touch left leg; REPEAT ON LEFT SIDE	for your waist and stomach	20	med.	23	fast	max you can do in 30 sec	fast
SITTING TUCKS—sit on deck and raise legs, tuck in, and straighten, don't touch deck.	for your stomach muscles	20	slow	23	med.	max you can do in 30 sec	fast
PUSH-UPS	arms	15	slow	18	med.	20	fast
RUNNING-IN PLACE, lift legs high	wind	2 min.	slow	2 min.	med.	2 min.	fast

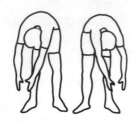

STRETCHER

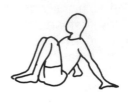

SITTING TUCKS

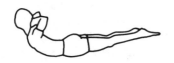

LOWER BACK EXERCISE

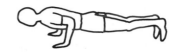

PUSH-UPS

SIT-UPS

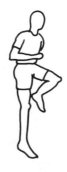

RUNNING-IN-PLACE

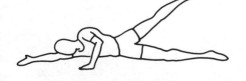

TRUNK MUSCLE EXERCISE

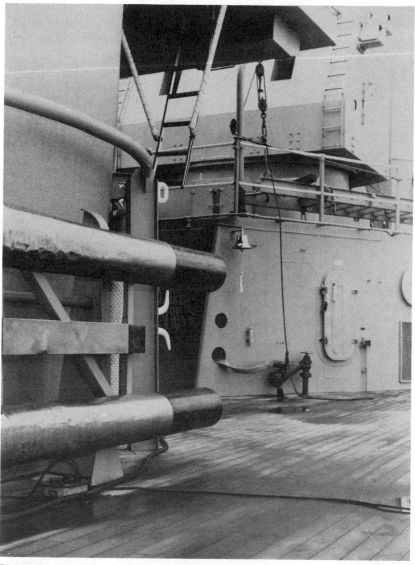

Photo 1.

The space shown in Photograph 1 is aboard a cruiser. Photos 2 and 3 illustrate how such space might be used for workouts.

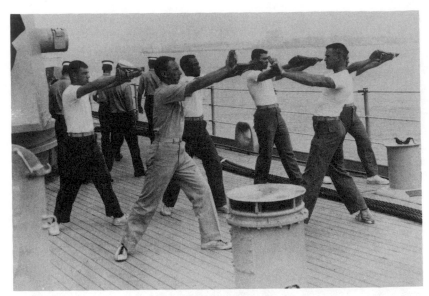

Photo 2.

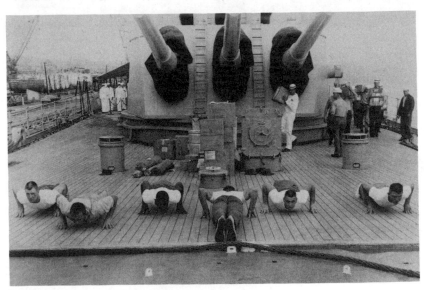

Photo 3.

Shown in Photographs 2 and 3 are Marines who are maintaining adequate levels of physical fitness. Marines seldom have a problem, because fitness is a prerequisite to survive in battle. As one can see, large ships provide space to carry out routine training programs.

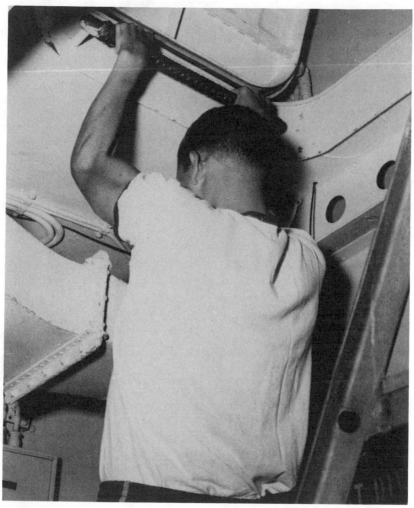

Photo 4.

It is an established fact that pull-ups are an excellent means of maintaining and increasing upper-torso strength. Photograph 4 illustrates a space suitable for this exercise. Good locations do exist aboard ship—however, one must consider if the space selected is a passageway, and if so, how busy it is and what the consequences might be from using the particular location for exercising. And obviously, if pull-ups are performed on a pipe not meant to support a 200-pound sailor, damage or injury could result.

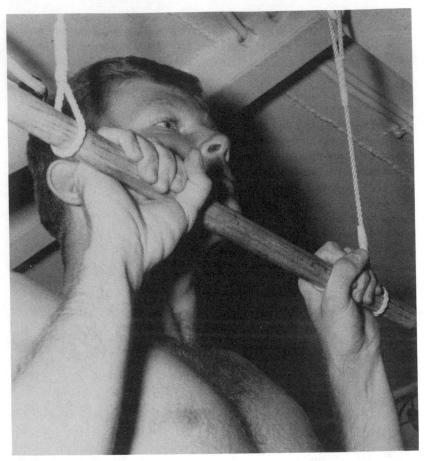

Photo 5.

Photograph 5 illustrates how one may use line to attach a wooden stick to the overhead, so that pull-ups can be done away from the main traffic patterns of the ship.

When taking exercise equipment to sea, it is important to consider the amount of room the package itself requires. Commercial devices are available that can be taken to sea.

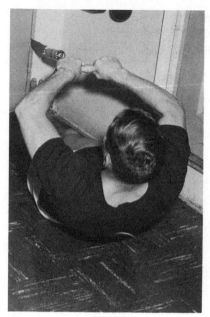 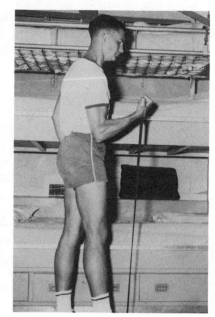

Photo 6.   **Photo 7.**

Photo 6 shows an Exergenie, which was an exercise device popular some years ago. In Photo 7 an exercise strap is used by a midshipman aboard ship. Both of these devices require small storage spaces and can be used effectively in training—however, special exercise devices are not really essential to train, as can be seen from following the program. It was designed for an aircraft carrier and successfully implemented not only by midshipmen, but by the ship's company as well.

Circuit training on an aircraft carrier

General description Ten exercise stations were designated on the forecastle, as shown. One man is positioned at each station, and a different exercise is executed at each one. Each exercise is carried out for fifteen seconds; each movement is repeated as rapidly as is practical. At the conclusion of each fifteen-second period, each man moves from his station to the next one within five seconds, and at the conclusion of 200 seconds—or 3 minutes and 20 seconds—all ten men have moved around all ten stations and have executed all ten exercises.

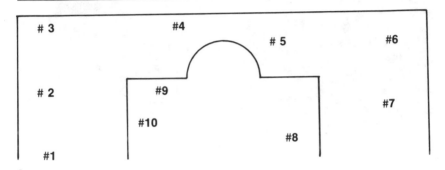

Specific exercises.
#1 Press overhead 40 lbs., plus bar.
#2 Overhand grip, full hang from stanchion.
   Lift legs to right angle from upper torso.
#3 Lateral raises with 5-pound weight in each hand.
#4 Run in place. Lift knees high.
#5 Pull-ups on bar welded to secondary connection.
#6 Step up and down on bench, 10-lb. weight in each hand.
#7 Climb rope fastened to flight deck.
#8 Sit on deck with a 5-foot bar across shoulders. Twist upper torso.
#9 Push-ups.
#10 Sit-ups with 5-pound weight held behind head.

Conclusion: These ten exercises are designed to maintain strength and endurance fitness. It is possible to provide activity for 50 men in 16 minutes and 10 seconds. It is possible to increase the exercise time at each station, and to increase the weight loads at stations 1, 3, 6, 8, and 10.

Four of the stations are pictured here.

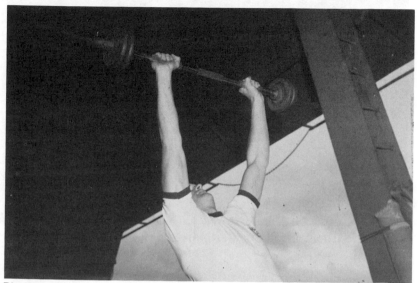

Photo 8. Station # 1: Overhead press, 40 lbs and bar

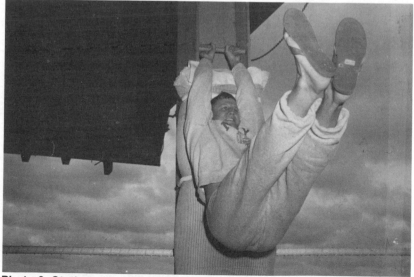

Photo 9. Station # 2: Leg-lift from a stanchion

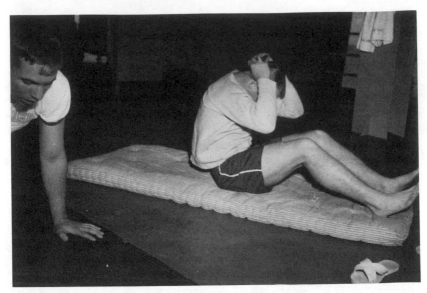

Photo 10. Station #9 and #10: Push-ups and sit-ups

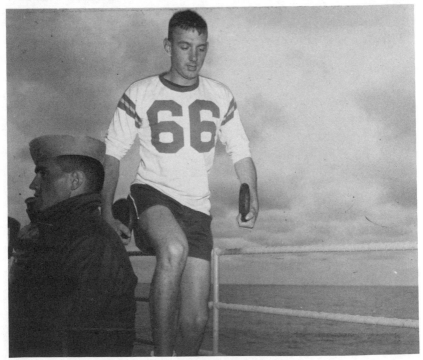

Photo 11. Station # 6: Stepping up and down with weight

Often old matresses can be used aboard ship to prevent abrasive contact with a steel deck or steel stanchion.

Such a circuit can be designed on many large ships, provided the commanding officer approves. There is no question that physical fitness problems on large ships can be solved, frequently in a unique manner.

This was the case on an aircraft carrier. A weight-lifting club had been established. The members had found a space topside, protected from the weather by the flightdeck. The sailors had constructed their own weights.

From the pipe shop they had been able to obtain stock steel to which pipe flanges were attached with vise grips. Thus it was easy to change the size of the pipe flanges. Each pipe flange had been taken to the ship's laundry where they had used the scales to determine the exact weight of each pipe flange. The weight was written on each flange in small numbers with paint. This illustrates how easily equipment problems might be solved when knowledge and resources are available. Physical fitness problems can also be solved on smaller ships.

Destroyers and frigates

The practical fitness program described previously was designed for a destroyer. However, a program of much greater depth was designed and implemented on that same destroyer as well.

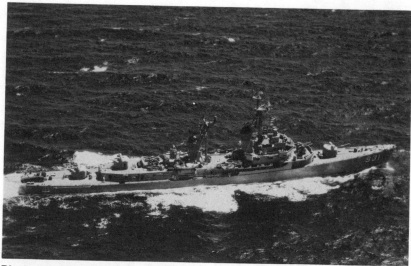

Photo 12. USS Forest Sherman

It was decided to install a series of exercise stations that could be combined for circuit training. The most suitable location was the torpedo deck. The exercise stations to be installed were essentially the same as those installed on the forecastle of the aircraft carrier. There was no difficulty in designating a space for each of the exercises.

The focal point of the circuit would be the mainmast of the ship, where a pull-up bar was welded. The exact location is indicated in Photo 13.

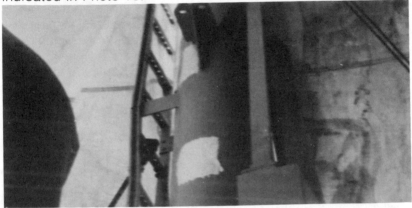

Photo 13: Pull-up bar location-mainmast

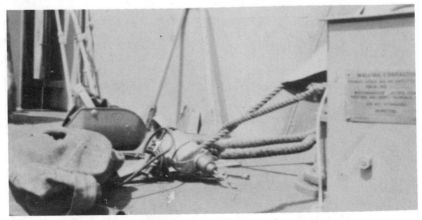

Photo 14: Pull-up bar ready for mounting

It was not difficult for the welding shop to manufacture the pull-up bar, shown in Photo 14, although the installation posed difficulties.

The destroyer was operating at a speed of over 30 knots. This meant that there was considerable wind topside—a weather condition not suitable for welding. When it became evident that the ship would not be slowing down for some time to come, a chief had the idea to rig a tent within which the welding could take place, shown in Photograph 15. Photo 16 shows the final installation phase.

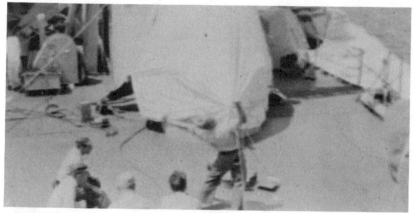

Photo 15: A tent was rigged for welding

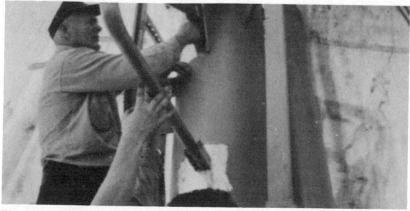

Photo 16: The pull-up bar is almost in place

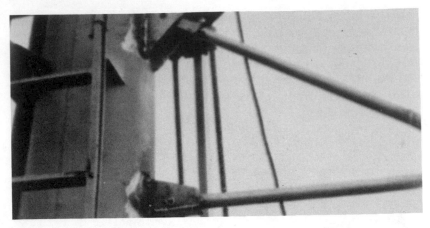

Photo 17: The pull-up bar is up

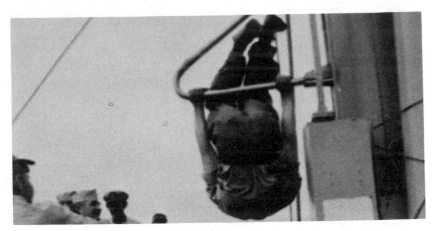

Photo 18: The pull-up bar is tested

Photos 17 and 18 show the final product and the initial stress test. There was no queston about it—the pull-up bar was installed.

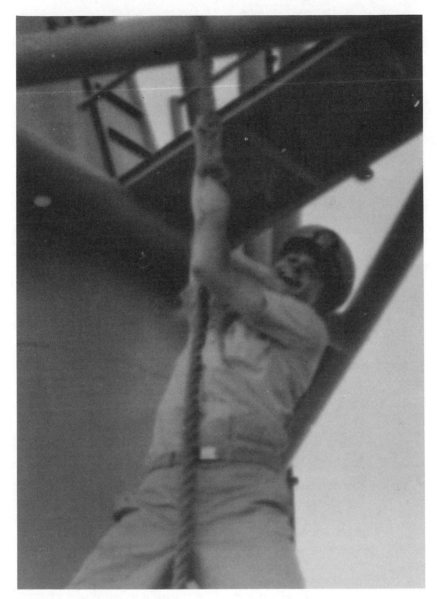

Photo 19: The climbing rope

A cross-section leading from the mainmast to the stack was used for the installation of the climbing rope, shown in Photo 19.

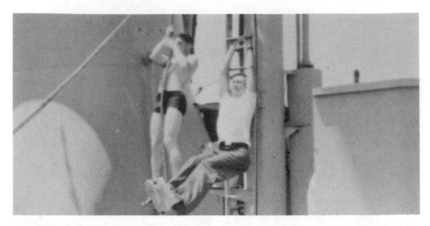

Photo 20: Use of ladder for abdominal exercises

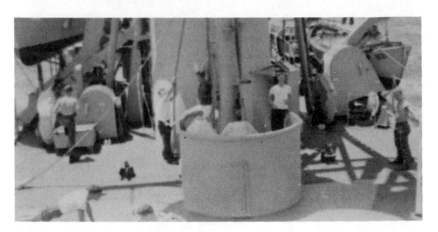

Photo 21: Circuit training stations

Photo 20 shows the station for leg raises, performed on a ladder adjacent to the climbing rope. In Photo 21 several training stations can be identified. Push-ups are done in front; further aft is the stepping station; to his right is the rope climb, followed by leg raises. Next can be seen a man who is about to jump up to begin pull-ups.

Not only did midshipmen use this circuit, but more and more members of the ship's company began to work out on the deck of this ship. The experiment was successful. A comparable circuit can be laid out on any destroyer or frigate.

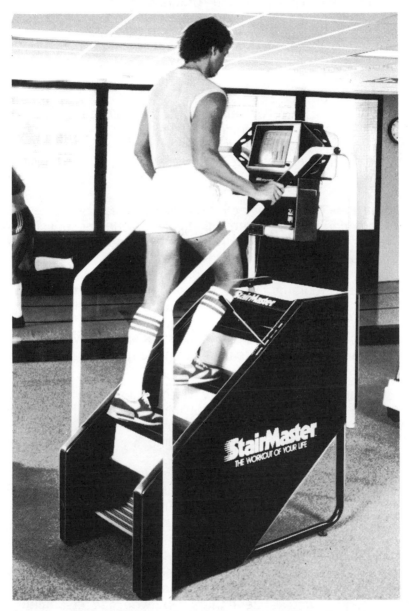

While it may be far more satisfying to maintain cardiovascular fitness by jogging, swimming, cycling or certain competitive games, it may be necessary while at sea to engage in alternate activities.

At the outset of this chapter, program #1 was described. The purpose of this program is to establish a foundation in physical fitness for untrained personnel at sea. Program # 2, described and illustrated in the chapter dealing with cardiovascular fitness, can be carried out aboard any ship. If personnel have a chair available in their quarters, the training can be carried out in the smallest of spaces.

While it is far more satisfying to maintain cardiovascular (aerobic) fitness by jogging, swimming, cycling, or certain competitive games, it may be neccesary while at sea to carry out the training routine described in program # 2.

Submarines Many of the activities described can be carried out on submarines, but there are limitations. It is often not possible to exceed certain noise levels. Thus, the exercise routines require precautions not needed on surface vessels.

On submarines it is possible to train for strength and endurance. Programs 1 and 2 described can be carried out, but with specific adaptations. Submarines, as well as other ships of the Navy, often have commercial weight training equipment aboard and submarines often provide stationary bicycles for the crew. Training methods are no different from those used ashore, as discussed in other sections of this book.

It makes little sense for naval personnel to train vigorously only when ashore. There is no such thing as a deposit in the bank of physical fitness. Training has to be continued while on deployment, not only for physical readiness, but also to maintain mental alertness and manage stress.

While stress management has been discussed in other parts of this book, it is pertinent to consider the following, published by the President's Council on Physical Fitness:

"Habitual exercisers show similar personality traits. After retesting 75 males who had formerly belonged to a fitness program, it was found that those subjects who had continued to exercise regularly proved to be less tense and frustrated, more tough-minded and prudent than men who had discontinued exercise".[4]

REFERENCES

1. McGinley II, E.S. "Preventing the Preventable Accident," *U.S. Naval Institute Proceedings*, June 1973, Vol. 99 (6), pp. 56-65.
2. United States Navy, Bureau of Naval Personnel. *BUPERSINST. 6100.2*, 30 August 1961.
3. United States Navy, Office of the Chief of Naval Operations. OPNAVINST 6110.1A, 15 August 1982.
4. President's Council on Physical Fitness and Sports. *Physical Fitness Research Digest*, Series 2, No.2, April 1972.

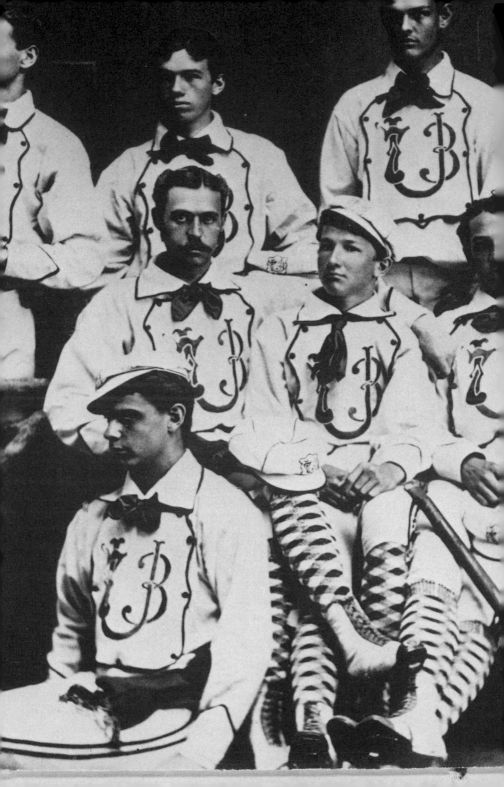

PART III

FITNESS IN SPECIAL SETTINGS

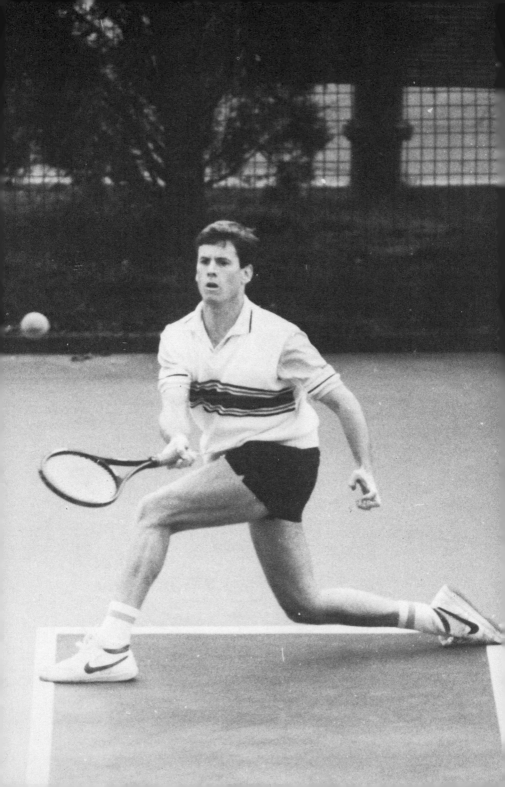

12

LIFETIME FITNESS FOR ADULTS

To die "young" as old as possible, attain a high degree of physical fitness and maintain it.

—HWL

OBJECTIVES

- Demonstrate the need to organize programs for adults because of the increased populations of older citizens.
- Describe the difference between chronological aging and physiological aging. Emphasize the documented changes as a result of deterioration of levels of physical fitness.
- Illustrate that personal lifestyle, rather than aging, brings forth degenerative diseases.
- Identify the leading causes of death.
- Review the literature that show how physical activity enhances health.
- Present a model of a physical fitness club to enable students to organize comparable clubs within military commands.
- Identify resource materials required if the physical fitness club is to be effective and permanent in nature.

INTRODUCTION

The number of people who will be 65 years of age and older will continue to increase throughout the coming decades. Statistics support this fact quite clearly.

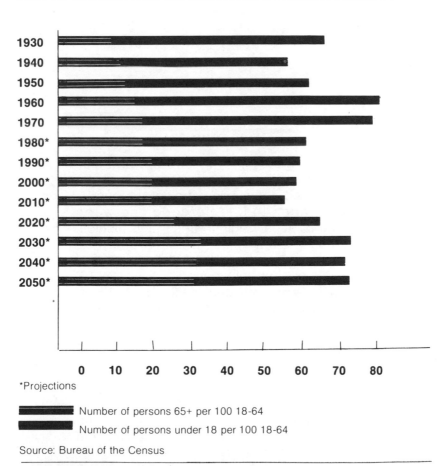

*Projections

Number of persons 65+ per 100 18-64

Number of persons under 18 per 100 18-64

Source: Bureau of the Census

Number of Persons Aged 65 and older and Under 18 per 100 Persons Aged 18-64. 1930-1980, and Projections to 2050

It is predicted that there will be 29 million Americans over 65 years of age by the year 2000. The well-being of such a large part of the American populaton will become increasingly more important throughout the coming decades. Well-being of the aged has been extensively investigated, and has been shown to be strongly related to health, socio-economic factors and degree of social interactions.[1], [2], [3] It appears, as Larson has stated, there is soundness in the folk wisdom, that health, wealth and love are the basis of happiness.

As one searches the literature, it becomes clear that health is consistently stated as a factor of primary importance. It is also evident that authors are more concerned with the curing of diseases than with their prevention. While the curing aspect is important, it has been clearly documented by professionals in the health and physical education fields, and by the President's Council on Physical Fitness that prevention of the deterioration of one's health is to a great extent in the hands of the individual.

THE PROCESS OF AGING

It is imortant to be able to distinguish between chronological aging and physiological aging. A pioneer in the investigation of the prevention of physiological aging is T.K. Cureton,[4] whose work has been published by the President's Council on Physical Fitness. Cureton explains that physiological aging is the gradual loss of physical powers and capacities after their gradual buildup to age 17. The plateau extends from 17 to 26. The decline begins as an average about 26 years of age. "Middle age" may be defined as the 26-65 age span, during which there is a steady loss of various powers and abilities. The 66-plus range is generally considered "old age." Research indicates, however, that chronological age is an unsatisfactory means of classifying men and women. Actual measures of functional fitness are a better indication of the degree of integration between the mind and the body.

Cureton[4] describes a study of 1000 adults from 50 cities. The curves of 60 fitness tests go steadily downward after 25 years of age. Physical tests in which a marked decline is recorded include: 1) accumulation of fat; 2) lowering of basal metabolic rates; 3) loss of muscular strength; 4) slowing of reaction time; 5) reduction in muscular endurance, muscular power, flexibility, balance and agility; 6) reduction in aerobic capacity; 7) an increase in ligamentous injuries and dislocation strains in the shoulders, knees and back; 8) increase in blood pressure and levels of cholesterol; and 9) a loss of capacity to adjust to intensive speed work or stress suddenly imposed.

All of these losses add up to physiological aging. In view of the fact that each of these areas can be controlled through proper physical activity, and personal lifestyle, it should be evident that chronological aging has little to do with the deterioration of the human organism.

PERSONAL LIFESTYLE:

In 1976, when our nation celebrated its 200th birthday, George F. Will in *Newsweek* (April 19, 1976)[5] stated that the American people were at least a billion pounds overweight. Will attributes this condition to the nation's favorite drugs—alcoholic beverages. In 1975 Americans consumed 621 million gallons of wine and distilled spirits, and the equivalent of 49 billion 12-ounce bottles of beer. In additoin to that, American men smoked 8.7 billion cigars and, all Americans combined smoked 600 billion cigarettes. Women and teenagers are smoking more than ever before. Statistics reveal that the lung cancer death rate among women tripled from 1962 through 1976.

STILL NUMBER ONE

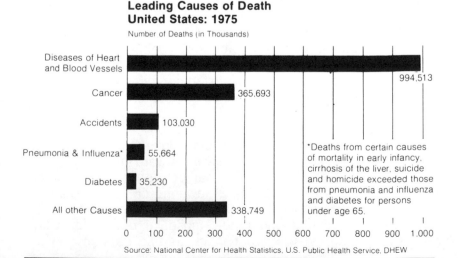

**Leading Causes of Death
United States: 1975**

Number of Deaths (in Thousands)

Diseases of Heart and Blood Vessels	994,513
Cancer	365,693
Accidents	103,030
Pneumonia & Influenza*	55,664
Diabetes	35,230
All other Causes	338,749

0   100   200   300   400   500   600   700   800   900   1,000

*Deaths from certain causes of mortality in early infancy, cirrhosis of the liver, suicide and homicide exceeded those from pneumonia and influenza and diabetes for persons under age 65.

Source: National Center for Health Statistics, U.S. Public Health Service, DHEW

Fortunately the picture is not entirely pessimistic. On November 14, 1980, on the *Today* show, Dr. Robert Levy, a cardiologist, reported that there was a 25 percent reduction in cardiovascular disease from 1968 to 1978. Dr. Theodore Cooper, a former Assistant Secretary for Health, observed the same trend as early as March 1977[6] when he stated, "The incidence of fatal heart disease has decreased by about 14% among Americans." Cooper said three factors contributed to the improved heart health: better dietary habits, less smoking and more exercise. He noted that the most significant change was in exercise habits.

In November 1982 the President's Council on Physical Fitness and Sports[7] reported the results of a *Washington Post-ABC News Poll* which stated that 53 percent of U.S. Adults exercise every day. While this figure is the highest of its kind, it is not out of line with other poll results. The Gallup Leisure Activities Index, which is generally considered to be one of the more reliable polls, reported a participation figure of 24 percent in 1961 and recently reported figures as high as 47 percent.

Whether these figures are completely accurate is less important than the fact that there is a definite trend toward increased physical activity for the sake of physical fitness on the part of the American people. Fortunately this trend is supported by increasing evidence which indicates that proper physical fitness training contributes significantly to the control of degenerative diseases.

PHYSICAL ACTIVITY AS A MEANS TO ENHANCE HEALTH

In the *American Journal of Cardiology*, Fox and Skinner,[8] in 1964, reported that the value of physical activity as a means of preserving or enhancing health has had advocates for centuries.[7] In the dialogues of Plato, Timaeus speaks of his belief that the body "by moderate exercise reduces to order, according to their affinities, the particles and affections which are wandering about . . . ." Many centuries later, in 1854, William Stokes[9] wrote about the "treatment of fatty degeneration of the heart." The patient must "adopt early hours, and pursue a system of graduated muscular exercise; and, it will often happen that after perseverance in this system the patient will be enabled to take an amount of exercise with pleasure and advantage—."

Throughout the ensuing decades, a certain number of studies continued to indicate the beneficial aspects of physical activity. In 1953 Morris and associates[10] examined the status of coronary heart disease of 31,000 London Transport employees aged 35 to 64. It was presumed that conductors were physically more active than drivers. The age-adjusted incidence rate of coronary heart disease (CHD) was higher in the drivers than among the conductors of the London double-decker buses.

Other investigators from 1956 to 1964 [11-17] compared active and sedentary populations in great detail. Time and time again it was found that more active segments of populations had a more favorable experience than those who lived a more sedentary life. Claims made for exercise have been supported by research. Physiologists have found that a systematic exercise program decreases stress and tension, helps prevent or cure the common backache, and provides a safeguard against gastrointestinal disorders such as ulcers and constipation. Evidence is beginning to emerge that exercise may even prevent cancer.

ORGANIZING A FITNESS PROGRAM

Many Americans are concerned because they know they have become increasingly physically unfit. The question of how to train older adults for a higher level of physical fitness is not easily answered.

Training becomes more difficult as physical deterioration becomes more manifest. The American public is inundated with advertisements which claim that conditioning can come about miraculously. This simply is not true. There are claims that isometrics provide the answer. Isometrics done correctly will enhance strength, but can do nothing for endurance; nor are sufficient calories used to have any impact on weight loss. Exercise devices are sold everywhere for various prices. "New" diets claim to bring about a desired level of physical fitness. This is not possible. There are no short cuts; crash methods will not work. It is most difficult to train alone for a higher level of physical fitness. If permanent progress is to be made, many principles must be rigidly followed. The inexperienced person must have patience, discipline, and competent guidance in his or her quest for physical fitness.

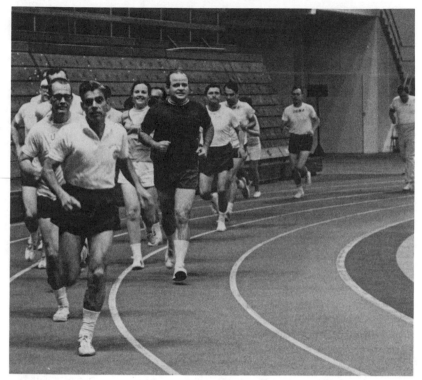

Author Heinz Lenz leads men's and women's jog.

USNA Adult fitness program If there are a number of people who seek improvement in their levels of physical fitness it is advisable to form a physical fitness club, under the auspices of the employer. A joint request should ask that a leader in adult physical fitness be provided for such a club. Precisely this occurred at the United States Naval Academy in 1967, when a large number of Academy faculty members decided that something had to be done about their lack of fitness.

Eight years later, in 1975, the program was published and described as follows. This description may well serve as an appropriate model in the organization of a fitness program.

Fifty officer and civilian faculty members and their wives met informally to engage in physical activities under professional guidance. The program is supervised by a member of the Naval Academy's Physical Education Department. Medical advice and guidance on nutrition are available to participants. Activities center primarily around cardiovascular training, designed to strengthen the heart. The exercises are geared to the level of physical fitness of the participants, beginning at a low level of stress. Periodically, tests and measurements are administered to evaluate progress. Training routines are scheduled Monday through Friday, with three days of participation per week considered adequate. The remaining two days are scheduled for convenience's sake because members have different schedules and are not always able to attend. Limited locker space, showers, towels, and clean athletic clothing are available. Participants must supply athletic shoes only.

Classroom session The first meeting of each season is scheduled in a classroom. Only in exceptional cases are new members admitted into the club after that organizational meeting. Initially, physical fitness and its component parts are defined. The purpose of the training sessions, increasing the level of cardiovascular fitness is emphasized.

Aerobic fitness All participants must realize that a cardiovascular training session lasts thirty minutes after a ten minute warmup phase. They must also watch for initial heart-beat intensities, which range from 130 heartbeats per minute to 155 heartbeats per minute. They must also be prepared to attend a minimum of three training sessions every week. Every member must understand that such a program will not bring about a loss of weight unless there is a distinct reduction of caloric intake. It is important, furthermore, for all to understand clearly that it is not possible to regain a high level of physical fitness in a short period of time and that the first 18 training sessions, the first six weeks, are little more than an adjustment period to physical stress.

Medical evaluation Another most important point which is stressed early in the program is that a routine of this nature should be undertaken only after the participant has had a physical examination. Experience has dictated that it is best if participants are given a blank form to present to their physician. In this manner, the physical examination is geared for an evaluation of the individual's ability to take part in the program without excessive risk. Naturally, it is easier for naval members to obtain a physical than for the civilian members. However, the importance of obtaining a proper physical examination is essential for all fitness program participants.

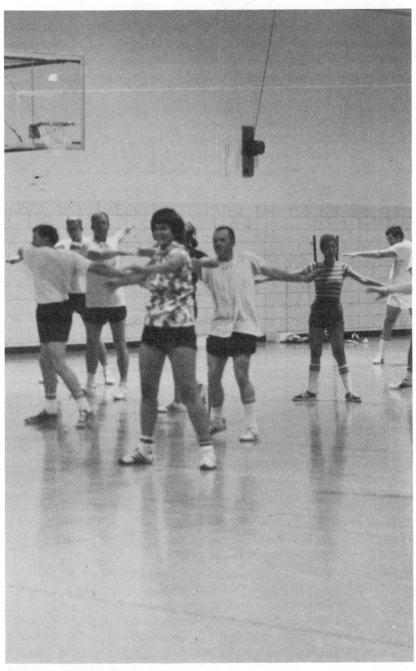

Aerobic exercise session

During the initial classroom orientation session, members fill out a record card with essential information: date of physical examination, weight, abdominal girth, resting heart rate, scores on a modified step test, scores on the five-minute step test, reclining blood pressure and more. Some entries are made at once, others periodically over the course of the program. The fact that physical fitness must not be competitive is emphasized at the initial meeting and throughout the training sessions.

Continuous rhythm exercises Fitness activities are patterned after the continuous rhythmical endurance program developed by T. K. Cureton, formerly of the University of Illinois. The participants exercise without pause at a changing pace. After the warmup, activities are intensified to lead to a point of fatigue, then the pace is reduced for recovery. In this manner—by stressing the cardiovascular system, relaxing, and then slowly building up to a point of fatigue—levels of cardiorespiratory fitness are increased. A roster of participating members is kept on the club bulletin board. Everyone checks his own attendance. Pertinent material is posted on the bulletin board, the assembly point before each training session. The members begin to know each other and enjoy working out as a group.

Muscular Fitness After adequate conditioning foundation is insured, the level of stress is increased. In addition, strength exercises such as push-ups and pull-ups are gradually introduced. Much guidance continues to be given verbally to the participants while the training goes on. Regularity is continually emphasized. Participants are encouraged to call any recurring pains to the attention of the leader. These can be corrected in some cases; in others, it may be simply a question of conditioning.

Facilities Even though the basic training routines are similar, the group works out in various locations. The group may work in an area surrounded by a 220-yard running track, or in an adjacent basketball court, in the hallways, up and down various stairs, or, when the weather is pleasant, at a large number of outdoor sites. The club members know that they will exercise outside only when shorts and a short-sleeve shirt are adequate cover.

When all activities of the club are considered, it becomes clear that any individual who wishes to train for physical fitness entirely on his own faces an almost insurmountable challenge.

IMPLEMENTING THE ADULT FITNESS PROGRAM

If the program is to be successful it requires not only enthusiastic leadership, but also a great deal of administration. Initially, the program must be publicized. This was done at the Naval Academy by the Deputy for Operations. The following notice was distributed to all faculty, officers and staff.

USANOTE 6100
12 September 1977

WHO: All Officers, civilian faculty members, enlisted personnel living on or working at the Naval Academy, staff members, and wives interested in participation.

WHAT: Group participation, under professional guidance, to improve cardiovascular endurance and muscle tone.

WHEN: Beginning 19 September 1977, there will be a mandatory organizational meeting for all old and new members. Regular classes will be held daily, except Saturday and Sunday, from 1210 to 1250.

WHERE: Field House, Open Area.

INFORMATION: The Physical Fitness Club will consist of a group of voluntary participants who will meet informally to engage in physical activities, under professional guidance. The program will be supervised by members of the Physical Education Department's Personal Conditioning Committee; medical advice will be available to participants.

The activities will be geared to the level of physical fitness of the participants. There will be a jogging program and an exercise program. The programs begin at a low level of stress. Periodical tests and measurements will be administered to evaluate progress.

Limited locker space, showers, towels and clean gear are available. Participants will need to bring gymnasium shoes only. There will be no charge.

ACTION: Complete attached registration form and send to Lynn Thomas, Field House, Stop 4A.

REGISTRATION

From: _____

(Last Name)   (First)   (Int)   (Rank)   (Dept)   (Ext)

To: Chairman, Personal Conditioning Committee, Physical Education Department

1. Please register me as a prospective member of the Physical Fitness Club. I am primarily interested in: (Check one)

    a. Jogging _____

    b. Exercises _____

At the organizational meeting the objectives and procedures are outlined. All who are interested are given the Health Examination Form. The date of the first training session is announced.

U S N A — PHYSICAL FITNESS CLUB

HEALTH EXAMINATION: To be performed by physician

NAME: _____ DATE _____
     Last   First   Init   PHONE_____
                                                Home

Address:_____
      Street   City   ZIP CODE

Normal	Abnormal		Please note details of abnormalities below
		Skin	
		Eyes	
		Ears	
		Nose	
		Throat	
		Mouth	
		Teeth	
		Thyroid	
		Heart	
		Lungs	
		Abdomen	
		Hernia	
		Feet	
		Rectal	
		Glandular	
		Reflexes	
		Ch. X-ray	
		Disability	

Laboratory work:

a. Urine sp. gr. ____ alb. ____ glucose ____ micro. ____

b. Complete blood count: Hbg.____ Hct.____ WBC____ Diff.____

c. ECG, 12 lead (copy, if available) _____

d. Blood pressure, syst.____disat.____e. cholesterol____mg.%____

f. Triglycerides____mg.%

Impression, remarks, recommendations: _____

The above person is capable of participating in a mild exercise program under the expert guidance of a competent, well trained physical educator who is a member of the physical education department of the United States Naval Academy.

Signed: _____ M.D.

Type, Name of Physician _____

Address _____

In case of illness or accident, permission is hereby given to arrange for emergency service:

Signed: _____

Physician to call_____

(Name)

                                                             (Phone)

NOTE: Return this form to JEANNIE CLARK HM 3, USN

FIELD HOUSE, USNA (Yard Mail Stop 4a)

USNA PHYSICAL FITNESS CLUB

	Sept				Oct											
	27	28	29	30	1	4	5	6	7	8	12	13	14	15	16	
Adams, Daniel B.																
Ammons, Paul F., LTjg																
Baker, Glenda																
Baker, Linda, D., DT3																
Bensinger, James L., MU1																
Brockus C. George, Asst Prof																
Brown, Donna K.																
Burns, Barbara, C.																
Cadell, Charles, E.																
Calisal, Sander, Asst Prof																
Carman, Ray A.																
Carroll, Candy M.																
Christopher, Billye R																
Clarke, Norman B., LCDR																
Cochran, Paul R., LT																
Corey, Suzane S.																
Costello, Wendy W																
Cox, Jay S., CAPT																
Cronyn, Lynne D.																
Crowley, Brenda E.																
Crowley, Fred R., MAJ																
Cunha, George, LCDR																
Davis, Katherine																
Davis, Richard L., Asst Prof																
Donnelly, Missy, LCDR																
Edelhoff, Marianne M.																
Ervin, Beverly A.																
Evans, Mary Sheila																
Evans, Phyllis D.																
Finster, George D.																
Fitzgerald, John D., Assoc Prof																

After the organizational meeting a roster is prepared from the names of those who attended. The roster is posted on a bulletin board where the members gather for their training sessions.

For each club member a five-by-seven card is prepared. Participants keep their respective cards up to date. The entries are made when appropriate.

USNA-Physical Fitness Club

	Last Name	First	Middle Init	Age	Rank	Dep't	Phone
Dates							
Pre-Physical							
Abdominal Girth							
Tricep Fat (mm)							
Weight							
Resting Heart Rate							
Step 60″, Rest 30″ Pulse Count/30″							
5′ Test & Cooper's Category							
Recl. Blood Press.							
Calories Req./24 Hrs							

On the club bulletin board information is posted so that the members can see how their performance is compared to national norms and scores of others in the Faculty Fitness Club.

Throughout the academic year, nutritional information is made available to the members. Once each semester the members attend a lecture by a sports medicine physician and nutritionist. Lectures are scheduled on regular training days at the training site.

Information made available is shown on the following pages.

USNA FACULTY PHYSICAL FITNESS CLUB

SATURATED FAT CONTENT OF FOODS

I Baked Goods
Bread, cakes (sponge, angel), crackers, doughnuts, macaroni, egg noodles, pretzels, rolls—*low* in saturated fat

II Cereals—*low* in saturated fats

III Dairy Products:
—Butter—*high* in saturated fat
—Buttermilk—*low* in saturated fat
—Cheeses—*high* in saturated fat *except* cottage cheese
—Cream—light or heavy—*high* in saturated fat
—Milk—*low* in saturated fat
—Ice cream—*low-moderate* in saturated fat
—Sherbet and yogurt—*low* to *moderate* in saturated fat
—Lard—*high* in saturated fat
—Margarine—*moderate* in saturated fat. Only *one-third* as much as butter, and it is preferred as a spread.

IV Oils
Coconut oil—very *high* in saturated fat. All other oils, such as corn oil and safflower oil are low in saturated fat, having *one-half* the amount of an equal amount of lard.

V Shortening such as Crisco and lard—*high* in saturated fat. Best shortenings are oils and margarine.

VI All fish products are *low* in saturated fat.

VII All flour products, such as barley, rice, oatmeal and corn meal, are *low* in saturated fats.

VIII All fruits are *low* in saturated fat.

IX Meats
Beef Products—*high* in saturated fat
Lamb Products—*high* in saturated fat
Pork Products—*high* in saturated fat
Rabbit & Veal—*low* in saturated fat
Poultry—*low* in saturated fat

X Nuts, except coconuts, are *low* in saturated fat.

XI Salad Dressing
Italian, French—*low* in saturated fat. Mayonnaise recipes & cheese recipes are moderate to *high* in saturated fat.

XII Brain, heart, kidney, liver—*low* in saturated fat.

XIII Sausages—*moderate* in saturated fat; *salami* however, has a *high* saturated fat content.

XIV All candies & vegetables are *low* in saturated fat.

XV Snacks—potato chips & similar products have a *moderate* to *high* saturated fat content, depending on how hard they are.

PHYSICAL FITNESS CLUB—USNA
LOW ANIMAL FAT DIET*

The principle of this diet is to substitute a vegetable (unsaturated) fat for animal (saturated) fat. Vegetable oils, such as Mazola (corn oil), should be used, Best Food Salad Oil (cottonseed), or safflower oils. These should be used in salad dressings and for cooking. The total amount eaten in a day should be 2 to 3 ounces. No oil or fat which is homogenized or hydrogenated should be eaten. Since this process changes an unsaturated fat to a standard one, the diet is not a reduction one, but can be used as such by the elimination of bread and potatoes. If underweight, use more of the unsaturated fatty acid oils, mixed in fruit juices.

EAT LESS

Cream, homogenized milk, whole milk

Ice cream
Soft or hard cheeses
Fried meats
Greasy gravies, greasy soups
Homogenized or hydrogenated peanut
  butter
Foods fried in deep fat, such as
  doughnuts and French-fried foods
Potato chips in cans
Pastries, particularly the
  French and Danish types

Pie and custards
Salad dressing not made of
  vegetable oil
Butter, oleomargarine, egg yolks
Chocolate
Liver and brain

EAT MORE

Skim milk, or defatted milk sub-
  stitute
Sherbets and ices, ice milk
Non-fat cottage cheese (not creamed)
Broiled meat, fish and fowl
Gravy substitute such as broth
Unhydrogenated peanut butter

Unsaturated vegetable oils for all
  frying (corn oil, etc.)
Potato chips only in paper bags
May have filling of fruit pie, but
  not crust unless it is made with
  vegetable oil
Angel food and sponge cake
Only Wesson oil, Mazola, Best
  Foods salad oil, etc.
Egg whites in cakes
Non-fat chocolate

SAMPLE MENU

Breakfast	*Lunch*	*Dinner*
Orange juice	Peach, non-fat cottage	Lean roast beef
Cereal with skim milk (sugar)	cheese	Scalloped potato (made
Toast-marmalade	Jello	with skim milk and
Coffee	Tea, coffee, skim milk	Mazola or Wesson Oil),
		string beans, stewed
		tomatoes, strawberry
		ice, tea, coffee

Survey Results

UNITED STATES NAVAL ACADEMY
Department of Physical Education
FACULTY PHYSICAL FITNESS

4 April 1973

From: Heinz Lenz
To: Faculty Fitness Participants
Subj: Training Sessions

1. Your performance on Cooper's twelve-minute test shows objectively that the physical fitness level attained by participants is "good."

2. Please answer the questions below to indicate your honest feelings.

3. I am suggesting that members not sign their names to get most a objective response:

1. I feel that our training sessions are:

(a) Too hard	(b) Not hard enough	(c) Fine
0	4	20

---

2. I would like to see more jogging in our program:

(a) Yes	(b) No	Don't care
10	13	1

---

3. I feel that our training sessions are begining to be boring:

(a) Yes	(b) No	Don't care
6	17	1

---

4. I am interested in:

(a) maintaining	(b) increasing my present level of physical fitness
10	15

---

5. I feel the program should continue along the same pattern as in past months:

(a) yes	(b) no
24	1

---

6. Optional comments:

"More variety of exercises" appears to be the response pattern on eight or nine of the ten or twelve comments.

UNITED STATES NAVAL ACADEMY
Department of Physical Education
PHYSICAL FITNESS CLUB

SUMMER PROGRAM

FREQUENCY: Work out three to four times a week. When away from the Annapolis area, be certain to work out at least twice a week. This is necessary to maintain the level of fitness you have now acquired. In middle age, after a 10 day "lay-off", a complete detraining period has taken place; don't let this happen. Maintain your investment.

WORK AREA: The Naval Academy Physical Education facilities are yours when areas are not needed for classes. To determine schedule, call ext. 2373 for Macdonough Hall or 2227 for the Field House.

Routine I — ANY PLACE, on athletic fields, in gymnasiums, at the beach, at home, in hotel rooms, in China, Japan or Russia. When you cannot jog, run in place or step up and down a chair.

Routine II —In Annapolis, Macdonough Hall or Field House. Away, in YMCA's, other universities, or use Routine I.

INSTRUCTIONS: Remember the basic principle of training. Warm up for a period of 10-15 minutes. Gradually increase the pace until you reach a level of fatigue, then ease off for a recovery. Again, gradually increase the pace. Stress and relax, stress and relax. Finally, taper off.

Routine I
Time periods: 30-40 minutes. Initially do each exercise 20 seconds; increase time periods if you so desire.
Warm up: The 10-15 minute warmup period is included in Routine I.

Routine II
Time periods: Low gear 20-25 min.
Medium gear 30-35 min.
High gear 40-45 min.
Warm up: Warmup period is not included in Routine II; Make up your own.

RECORD KEEPING: 1. Know how many workouts you have completed by September.
2. To measure progress for Routine II, apply point system periodically.
*****

As a result of the training sessions, the members are familiar with Routines I & II and the point system, based on Cooper.

United States Naval Academy
Department of Physical Education
Faculty Fitness 1976-1977

Routine I

Note: Work out a minimum of three times a week. Always warm up for at least ten minutes as we did in class. Remember to taper off by walking.

Endurance workout
Bend and twist
Arm circles   45 sec.
Crawl forward and back
Butterfly
Jog and sprint, stepping, straddle hopping, etc.   2 min.
Alternate leg kicks   60 sec.
Side leg raises
Flutter front and behind   30 sec.
Down twice, up on toes and reach   60 sec.
Jog and sprint, stepping, straddle hopping, etc.   2 min.
Grasp biceps, bend forward way down, hold 10-12 sec.
Grasp hips, feet shoulder width, bend backward, way back
Rock, hands behind neck, arch way up   30 sec.
Straddle hopping, scissors, bouncing   30 sec.
Deep breathers for recovery
Flexibility to the right and left, hold 10-12 sec.
Sitting tucks
Bicycle position (three-way stretch)
Push-up, 15-25 reps
Bicycle position, extend feet and hands to rear, 30 reps
Sit-ups, 15-25 reps
Sitting, soles, heels touching, grasp toes, bounce knees

Remember: *Intensity* (125 b/m-140 b/m) *duration*—30 minutes after ten-minute warmup; *frequency*—three times per week, preferably four times per week.

ROUTINE II

	LOW GEAR	MEDIUM GEAR	HIGH GEAR
Jogging	1 lap	1 lap	1 lap
Arm Circles (Reverse halfway through)	30	50	70
Forward Bending	10	20	30
Side Bending (Reverse halfway through)	20	30	40
Rope (Use chalk)	10 pulls	climb 10'	climb 20'
Run Backwards	1 lap	1 lap	1 lap
Run side straddle hop—face in	½ lap	1 lap	2 laps
Run side straddle hop—face out	¼ lap	1 lap	2 laps
Deep breathers	5	7	10
Sit-ups, knees bent	10	20	30
Univ. gym leg press (body weight)	5	10	20
Chin-ups	2	3	8
Run full speed	1	1½	2
Forced breathers and walk one-half lap	2	4	6
Dips on parallel bars	2	5	10
Scissors on back	25	50	100
Weights: upright rowing	8	10	15
Standing broad jump for distance on mats	4	8	10
Run 3/4 speed	1 lap	2 laps	3 laps
Deep breathers	2	4	6
Univ. gym curls—one-quarter body weight	5	10	15
Front rolls, on mat	2	3	6
Side leg raises, right and left	10	15	30
Run in place, knees, heels, toes high	50 steps	100 steps	150 steps
Push-ups	5	10	20
Back-arching	5	10	15
Straddle-hops	10	20	30
Univ. gym bench press 1/3 body weight	5	10	15
Bench stepping	50	100	150
Weights-military press	10	20	30
Run-laps	2	4	8

The purpose of the inclusion of material is to show those aspects of physical fitness which must be included in any adult physical fitness training program. The model described was successful and of benefit to a large portion of the Naval Academy community.

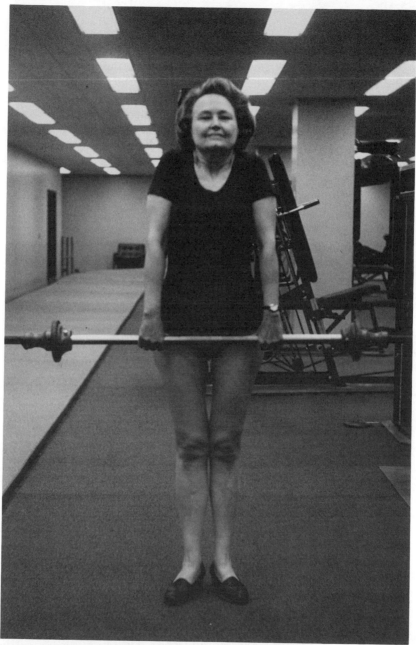

An effective adult physical fitness program will include activities to develop muscular fitness.

REFERENCES

1. Fox, J. H. "Effects of Retirement and Former Work Life on Women's Adaptation in Old Age." *Journal of Gerontology,* 1977, 32(2), pp.196 - 297.
2. George, L. K. and Maddox, G. L. "Subjective Adaptation to Loss of the Work Role: A Longitudinal Study." *Journal of Gerontology, 1977, 32(4), pp. 456 - 462.*
3. Larson, R. *"Thirty Years of Research on the Subjective Well-Being of Older Americans."* Journal of Gerontology, 1978, 33(1), pp. 109 - 125.
4. Cureton, T. K. "The Value of Exercise for Fitness and Health." *Physical Fitness Research Digest,* July 1971, President's Council on Physical Fitness and Sports, Washington, DC 20210, pp. 7 - 10.
5. Will, George F. "Run for Your Life." *Newsweek,* 9 April, 1976, p. 100.
6. President's Council on Physical Fitness and Sports. *Newsletter,* March 1977, p. 7.
7. President's Council on Physical Fitness and Sports, Newsletter, November 1982, p. 11.
8. Fox, S. M. and Skinner, J. S. "Physical Activity and Cardiovascular Health." *American Journal of Cardiology,* December 1964, 14(6), pp. 731-746.
9. Stokes, W. *Diseases of the Heart and Aorta,* Dublin: Hodges and Smith, 1854, p. 357.
10. Morris, J., Heady, J., Raffle, P., Roberts, C., and Parks, J. "Coronary-heart Disease and Physical Activity of Work," *Lancet,* 1953, 2(1053).
11. Stamler, J. et al.,"Prevalence and incidence of coronary heart disease in strata of the labor force of a Chicago industrial corporation." *Journal of Chronic Disease,* 11: 405, 1960.
12. Breslow, L. and Buell, P. "Mortality from coronary heart disease and physical activity of work in California." *Journal of Chronic Diseases,* 11: 421, 1960.
13. Brunner, D. and Manelis, G. "Myocardial infarction among members of communal settlements in Israel." *Lancet,* 2: 1049, 1960.
14. Karvonen, M. "Physical activity, cholesterol metabolism and atherosclerosis." *Schweizer Zeitschrift der Sportsmedizin,* 9: 1, 1961.

15. Taylor, H. L. et al., "Death rates among physically active and sedentary employees of the railroad industry." *American Journal of Public Health*, 52: 1697, 1962.
16. Brozek, J., Kihlberg, J., Taylor, H. L. and Keys, A. "Skinfold distributions in middle-aged American men: A contribution to norms of leanness-fatness." *Annals of the New York Academy of Science*, 110: 492, 1963.
17. Kahn, H. "The relationship of reported coronary heart disease mortality to physical activity of work." *American Journal of Public Health*, 53: 1058, 1963.

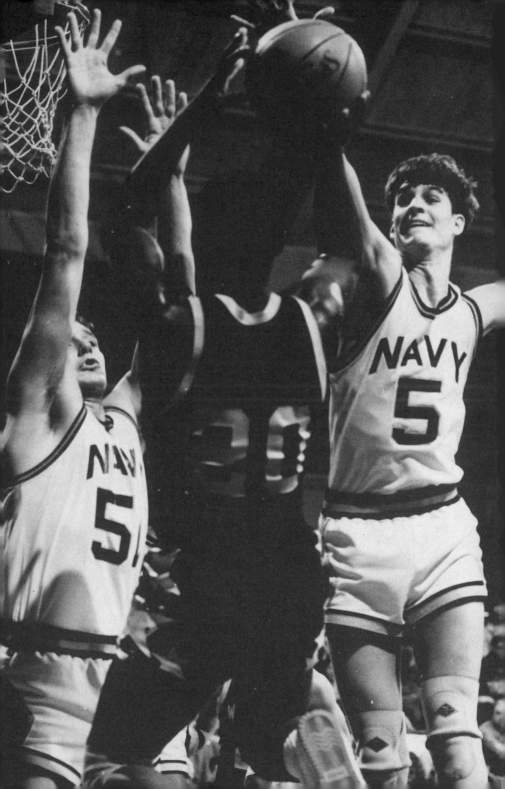

13

SPORTS FITNESS . . . FIT FOR SPORTS

I wish to preach, not the doctrine of ignoble ease, but the doctrine of the strenuous life.

—Theodore Roosevelt, 1899

OBJECTIVES

- Identify the reasons individuals select and play sports.
- List the major benefits of sports participation.
- Describe the opportunities for sports participation that are available to midshipmen.
- Discuss why some sports contribute to physical fitness and others do not.

AMERICA'S SPORT HERITAGE

Amateur and professional sports play a significant role in the lives of Americans. Given a rich sports heritage, excellent sports and recreational facilities, and the availability of individual resources, sports participation today spans a lifetime. Participation begins early in life and can continue well into the adult and senior years.

Improvement in sports equipment technology and the removal of many attitudinal barriers has also led to the recent inclusion of many handicapped and disabled persons in sports activities. In America sports are for everyone and nearly everyone is for sports.

In this chapter we will briefly examine the general reasons why people play sports, the benefits of sports involvement and the ways in which selected sports may contribute to physical fitness.

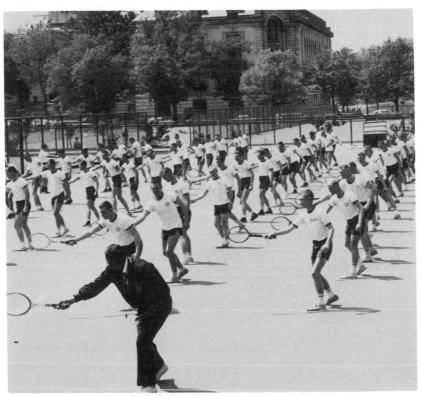

In America sports are for everyone and nearly everyone is for sports.

WHY PEOPLE PLAY SPORTS

There are many personal reasons people play sports, but in general most people do so for three reasons: 1) because sports provide an excellent means of recreation and relaxation; 2) because sports participation is a fun way to improve health and fitness; and 3) because people enjoy the competition that sports provide.

Recreation and relaxation For many individuals, sports participation can be a wholesome and life-enriching pursuit. It often leads to an expansion of social relationships as well. In addition, for those who do not take themselves too seriously, sports can serve as an excellent catharsis and have a therapeutic effect on mind and body. The release of muscular tensions during participation is frequently observed in individuals who consciously use sports as a tool for relaxation.

Physical fitness and health Recently in our society many individuals have begun to participate in sports for the health and fitness benefits. This perhaps has resulted from the media emphasis upon the degenerative illnesses that often result from sedentary and other poor lifestyle behaviors.

But do all sports contribute to the improvement of health and fitness? In certain sports a certain skill level must be achieved before we can reap the fitness benefits. On the other hand, if you do not have the minimal level of fitness you may not be able to become as proficient as you would like. Another question is whether the sports we select contribute to the specific fitness goals we desire. Later in this chapter we will examine which sports are most compatible with your personal fitness objectives, your psychological make-up and your physical capacities.

Competition Engaging in team or individual sports contests with other participants can be a fulfilling experience. Friendly sports competition, when kept in proper perspective, allows one to test his or her personal level of skill development and to strive toward individual excellence.

Competition often brings out the best in each of us. It pushes us to improved levels of skill and gives us a sense of personal accomplishment and success. For many people sports competition can be an ego-builder. Competition in sports can therefore act as a natural positive and constructive force that could carry over into our daily lives.

But sports competition can also have a negative side and can be a non-constructive element in our personal development. When we become obsessed with winning (especially at all costs), and when losing is taken out of its proper perspective, it can destroy our egos and our balanced sense of what is important to us. But for most enthusiastic sports competitors, participation fortunately does represent a fulfilling, refreshing and enjoyable experience that is repeated with regularity.

WHAT SPORTS DO FOR US

In the previous section we alluded to some of the general benefits of sports participation. At the U.S. Naval Academy sports participation is designed to develop other personal qualities as well as those already touched on. All these qualities are important to the military profession, and most are highly desirable for civilian sports participants as well.

Health and fitness Sports requiring physical effort, those which make demands upon our cardiovascular and muscular systems, contribute most to our health and physical fitness. Sports such as bowling, softball, and golf are recreational and relaxing, but not very fitness-stimulating—in fact, many people select them because they do not require strenuous effort.

Sports such as rowing, basketball, soccer and gymnastics generally promote fitness at a high level. One should remember that sports requiring a high level of skill do not automatically promote the health-related components of fitness. A sport such as basketball generally requires a good level of physical fitness as well as a fairly high level of proficiency.

At the Naval Academy, sports participation also fosters the other important qualities of military preparedness.

Self-discipline Improvement in self-discipline is one that everyone admires. Self-discipline enables us to use our abilities to our fullest potential and helps us fulfill our personal, social and occupational commitments responsibily.

Teamwork The development of cooperation skills and attitudes help us learn to be a team player, to view ourselves not only as an individual but also as an important part of the whole effort. This is important whether we are citizens who must share the responsibilities of the community or military professionals who must help maintain the integrity and effectiveness of our unit.

Sports can teach us to work closely and effectively with others for the common good.

Military preparedness Sports place physical and mental demands upon us and can teach us to be resourceful. In short, sports can help train and toughen us for those threats and tragedies which are unfortunately real in our lives. Civilian emergency preparedness can be an important outcome of sports participation.

At the Naval Academy a career officer's training must include the preparation for the severe tests of mental and physical endurance that may be encountered in a hostile military environment. Although no training ever prepares one perfectly for such events, intense sports competition comes close. All of the service academies have recognized this fact since their inception.

SPORTS FOR MIDSHIPMEN

As previously described sports participation is an integral and important element in the training of midshipmen. The requirements for participation are strict, and every midshipman must meet them prior to graduation.

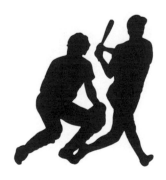

The following charts reflect the typical sports opportunities and the extent of participation available to midshipmen. Needless to say, such a program would not be possible without the organization, equipment and facilities of the Academy to implement such a program.

INTRAMURAL SPORTS PROGRAM PARTICIPATION

FALL
28 August–20 October

Sport	Participants	Teams	Contests
Basketball	540	36	147
Soccer	576	36	147
	1116		294
*Boxing	96	6	15
Crew	90	6	30
Cross Country	96	6	30
Fencing	72	6	15
*Football	198	6	30
Handball	90	6	30
Squash	72	6	30
Swimming	96	6	30
Tennis	90	6	30
*Wrestling	96	6	30
	996		270
Gymnastics	322	1 Meet	
Fall	150		
Fall Total	2294		565

WINTER
31 October–2 March

COMPANY SPORTS

Sport	Participants	Teams	Contests
Fieldball	720	36	147
Touch Football			
*Unlimited	684	36	147
*Lt. Weight	684	36	147
	2088		441

BATTALION SPORTS

	Participants	Teams	Contests
Handball	90	6	30
Squash	72	6	30
Team Handball	84	6	30
	246		90

WOMEN'S REGIMENTAL SPORTS

	Participants	Teams	Contests
Badminton	20	2	7

PROGRAM OFFICIALS

Winter	160	
Individual	86	

BRIGADE BOXING CHAMPIONSHIPS

NUMBER OF CONTESTS

	Participants	Teams	Contests
Winter Total	2600		538

SPRING
14 March–8 May

Sport	Participants	Teams	Contests
Softball			
Fast Pitch	576	36	147
Slow Pitch	576	36	147
Knockabout			
Racing	180	36	10 races
	1332		304
Basketball	90	6	30
*Rugby	198	6	15
Volleyball	90	6	30
*Lacrosse	120	6	30
Tennis	90	6	30
Track	156	6	15
Water Polo	84	6	30
Squash	72	6	30
Weightlifting	60	6	15
	960		225
Softball	36	2	7
Tennis	30	2	7
	66		14
Spring	146		
Spring Total	2504		543

VARSITY PROGRAM

FALL
28 August-20 October

	Maximum Squad
Cross Country	28
*Football	155
*Football (150 lb.)	80
Sailing (Men)	
Class A	40
Shields/Dinghy	51
Yawls	48
Sailing (Women)	
Shields/Dinghy	12
Soccer	60
Golf	17
Tennis	26
Volleyball	24
	541

WINTER
31 October-2 March

	Maximum Squad
Basketball (Men)	36
Basketball (Women)	24
Fencing (Men)	35
Fencing (Women)	24
Gymnastics	40
Pistol	23
Rifle	19
Squash	18
Swimming (Men)	40
Swimming (Women)	24
Track (Indoor)	75
*Wrestling	40
	398

SPRING
14 March-8 May

	Maximum Squad
Baseball	44
Crew (Hvywgt)	60
Crew (Ltwgt)	42
Crew (Women)	36
*Football	160
Golf	17
*Lacrosse	60
Sailing (Men)	
Class A	40
Shields/Dinghy	51
Yawls	48
Sailing (Women)	
Shields/Dinghy	12
Tennis	22
Track (Outdoor)	85
	677

OUT OF SEASON SPORTS

Sport	No.	Sport	No.	Sport	No.
Baseball	50	Baseball	50	Fencing	30
Crew (Men)	194	*Brigade Boxing	86	Gymnastics	55
Crew (Women)	36	Crew (Men)	194	Pistol	11
Fencing	30	Crew (Women)	36	Rifle	14
Golf	26	*Lacrosse	50	Soccer	35
Gymnastics	55	Tennis	12	Squash	10
*Lacrosse	110	TOTAL	428	Swimming	35
Pistol	17			*Wrestling	35
Rifle	20			TOTAL	225
Squash	30				
Swimming	35				
Tennis	26				
Track	65				
*Wrestling	55				
TOTAL	749	TOTAL	1132	TOTAL	1181

TOTAL 1555

*Male Midshipmen Only

PLEBE PROGRAM

Sport	No.	Sport	No.	Sport	No.
Cross Country	22	Basketball	25	Baseball	30
*Football	130	Fencing	35	Crew (Hvywght)	47
*Football (150 lb.)	33	Gymnastics	55	Crew (Ltwgt)	35
Sailing	30	Pistol	20	Golf	12
Soccer	50	Rifle	19	*Lacrosse	45
TOTAL	265	Squash	12	Sailing	30
		Swimming	40	Tennis	20
		Track (Indoor)	60	Track (Outdoor)	60
		*Wrestling	40	TOTAL	279
		TOTAL	306		

FITNESS BENEFITS OF SPORTS

It is common to overhear two individuals discussing the fitness merits of one sport over another. One person might express the view that he is fit because he swims for thirty minutes three days a week at the local YMCA. Another individual may state that she plays tennis for four hours every Saturday morning, which keeps her fit and thin. Some people may even think that participation in the Friday night bowling league or the Sunday softball league is an excellent way to maintain fitness.

If one of the primary reasons for participating in a sport is to develop or maintain a reasonable level of fitness, then how do we know whether we are getting enough of it to qualify? Just how are the fitness merits of recreational and competitive sports determined? Too often we use the subjective level of the tiredness we experience as the single criterion of benefit. Some individuals measure fitness by the degree of pain resulting from the activity. Actually, both of these factors tell you very little about the fitness merits of a sport. What you need to evaluate is whether the activity is of sufficient *intensity*, *duration* and frequency to cause physiological adaptations in your body. In other words, the exercise must produce a "training effect."

These factors are discussed thoroughly in the chapters on cardiovascular, muscular and flexibility fitness, but we will refresh your memory and review each of them briefly.

Cardiovascular fitness activities (aerobics) are relatively easy to evaluate. The questions to be answered, whether you are playing a singles game of racquetball or throwing a frisbee with a friend, are: 1) Does the activity stimulate the heart rate enough to reach the aerobic training zone, i.e. above sixty percent of one's maximum exercise capacity? 2) Does the heart rate remain in the training zone continuously at least fifteen minutes or longer? 3) Is the activity at this intensity and duration performed minimally three times per week?

Generally sports activities that fit the above criteria will produce a "training effect" and are sufficient to meet minimal levels of cardiovascular fitness. If you remain unsure whether you are getting enough aerobic exercise, you can maintain a fitness journal and keep track of your aerobics points using Dr. Kenneth Cooper's point charts. Remember that Cooper recommends thirty-five (35) points a week for men and twenty-seven (27) points a week for women.

By using one of the two above methods or both to assess sports for their aerobic fitness benefits, you will be able to settle most disputes regarding which activities provide the best fitness results. How the sport is played determines its fitness benefits, however. Two individuals may each play forty minutes of tennis singles and only one person may benefit with respect to fitness.

Muscular fitness benefits resulting from participating in a variety of sports is not as clear-cut as aerobic fitness. Participants initially must ask themselves three fundamental questions: 1) Do I currently have enough muscular strength or endurance to perform the sport activity at my desired level? 2) Will additional muscular strength or endurance help me perform the sport better than I am now performing it? 3) Will the sport help me increase my level of muscular strength or endurance if this is one of my personal fitness goals?

As you consider these questions, keep in mind that some sports may raise the level of muscular fitness in specific muscle groups at first, but as skill proficiency improves no further gains are evident. In this instance you may have to supplement your sports participation with weight training or other progressive resistance exercise if you desire to continue improving muscular fitness. Remember also that no two individuals gain muscular fitness at the same rate regardless of the similarity of the activity.

Usually a sport will provide gains in *muscular strength* (the ability to exert force with a single muscle contraction) if the movements are short, intense and are made against resistance. Wrestling, for example, is a sport which can greatly enhance muscular strength primarily because an opponent is often resisting a movement. The interior blocking lineman in football is another example of movement offered against a resistance (another lineman). Football is often considered a power activity— that is, it combines the elements of strength and speed.

Muscular endurance (the ability of a muscle or muscle groups to continue a local movement repeatedly without fatiguing) can also be developed in sports that offer resistance to the movement. Long-distance swimming is an excellent example of a sport where the water provides resistance while the swimmer must repeat arm stroking continuously for long periods.

A more accurate way to determine whether a sport has developed muscular fitness for you is to do a pre- and post-measure of these factors. Determine which muscle groups or movements are involved in your sport, and then test yourself with a set of weights. The maximum weight you can lift in a single exertion represents your present strength level. Then select a weight at about 40% of your maximum capacity and lift it repeatedly to the point of fatigue. Measure your improvement with the tests in about four to six weeks. If you prefer a more accurate and scientific method to measure these fitness factors, seek out a nearby sports medicine center or university center that will be willing to test you. Sometimes researchers are looking for subjects to use in such tests.

Flexibility fitness can be evaluated with respect to a given sport by observing whether the movements specific to the sport are performed at full range of motion. For example, did you know that a sprinter takes a running stride about twice as long as the long distance runner and may therefore have more flexibility in the same group of running muscles? Gymnastics requires and develops flexibility because of the movements required in that sport. As indicated in the chapter on flexibility, some sports may actually reduce flexibility in certain muscle groups. In addition to the tests of flexibility identified in this text, sequence photographs or video analysis of your participation can also indicate whether or not the sport is providing the degree of flexibility you desire from it. If it does not, then add some stretching exercises to your program.

Skill-related fitness elements are almost always improved through sports participation. Health-related elements or motor fitness factors are important to that sport and can carry over into other sports or aspects of our well-being, such as having good dynamic posture. As skill techniques improve, the neuro-muscular patterns improve to help you perform more effectively and efficiently. Improvements in coordination, reaction time, agility, balance, speed and power therefore mean greater economy of effort during participation, which allows you to play longer and enjoy it more.

SELECTING SPORTS AND FITNESS ACTIVITIES

We are indeed fortunate to live in a society where virtually unlimited opportunities exist to select and participate in fitness and sports activities. Whether you participate for relaxation, health, recreation, competition or to earn a living, a broad spectrum of sports opportunities is available to you. Although you may not have a specific reason for participating, you may wish to select activities you are likely to enjoy, which are suited to your abilities, and which will contribute to your general fitness level.

Select those activities from the activity list that you would like to try, discuss the activity with someone who is already participating in it, take basic instruction if desirable, but by all means—go for it!

Participate!

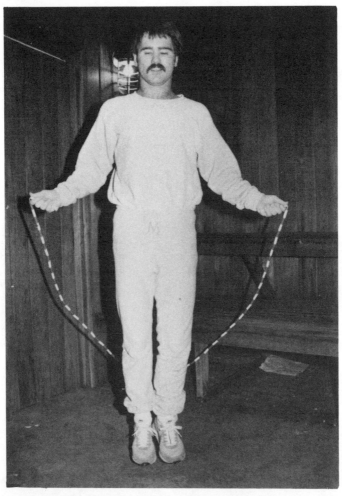

Select an activity that you would like to try and go for it!

SPORT/EXERCISE/ ACTIVITY!	FITNESS BENEFITS	PARTICIPATION DISADVANTAGES	PRECAUTIONS
Badminton Singles	Develops agility and coordination Excellent aerobics for skilled players	Need indoor court	
Doubles Recreational	Good for less active people Generally low fitness benefits Promotes relaxation	None: Can play anywhere	Teamwork is essential
Baseball	Except for pitcher/catcher has few fitness benefits	Need teams and field Requires excellent skills	Not recommended for older adults
Basketball	Excellent all around fitness activity when played full court		Should get into shape first
Bowling	Relaxation and recreational Low level of fitness development	Cost and facilities	Select proper weighted ball
Boxing	Excellent all around fitness activity	Requires intense training/head injuries	Not appropriate for most people
Canoeing (kayaking)	May develop upper body muscular endurance. Can be competitive or recreational	Equipment required	Wear life vests Helps to be a swimmer
Climbing (rock/mountain)	Develops muscular fitness, some aerobics	Special skills needed	Must be fit and trained
Crew	Excellent all around fitness development	Need special training and equipment	Get fit before competing
Cross Country Running	Mainly aerobic activity and leg endurance	Need special training	Run in safe areas

SPORT/EXERCISE/ ACTIVITY!	FITNESS BENEFITS	PARTICIPATION DISADVANTAGES	PRECAUTIONS
Cycling Single speed	Excellent for aerobics f follow training principles	Must have good balance	Other traffic
10-speed	Excellent aerobics if training principles followed Muscular leg endurance	Some training needed in shifting gears	Traffic/road conditions
Stationary	Excellent aerobics and leg endurance if training principles are followed	Equipment cost	none/relatively safe
Dancing Aerobics Ballet Ballroom Disco	All can be aerobic if training principles are followed, except ballroom (intensity too low)	Special training for ballet	Progress slowly/ most geared for all ages
Jazzercises Round Square Tap	All can be relaxing and reduce tension Some muscular endurance in lower body		
Fencing	Develops coordination, agility and muscular endurance with some aerobics	Special training required	Supervision required
Field Ball	Excellent all around fitness activity except for goalie	Physical contact injuries	Should be in condition before playing
Field Hockey	Excellent all around fitness sport except for goalie	Requires special stick skills/some injuries	
Football Touch	Relaxation/recreation with few fitness gains		Direct contact should be avoided
Flag	Muscular fitness with little aerobic benefits		Avoid if injury prone

SPORT/EXERCISE/ ACTIVITY!	FITNESS BENEFITS	PARTICIPATION DISADVANTAGES	PRECAUTIONS
Tackle	Little aerobic benefits with mainly muscular and skill fitness benefits	Special training and equipment required	Not for older adults Must be well supervised
Golf	Some aerobics if you walk and some flexibility when swinging	Course time/equipment	Lower back strain
Gymnastics	Mainly muscular fitness, agility, flexibility, coordination	Special facilities, coaching and training	Not advised for older adults
Hockey Ice	Excellent all around fitness activity, except for goalie	Good skater and need rink	Use protective equipment
Lacrosse	Excellent all around fitness sport, except for goalie	Special training/ equipment	Contact can cause injuries if unprotected
Martial Arts	Muscular fitness, coordination, and agility with possible aerobics (depends upon how long it is performed)	Special training required	Seek professional instruction
Racquetball	Good all around activity but may not be aerobic if played at recreational pace	Facilities and costs	Eye protection necessary
Rope Jumping	Excellent in all respects if training principles followed	May be too anaerobic for heart patients	Perform in large enough space
Rugby	Mainly muscular fitness with good aerobics when running continuously	Possible injuries due to lack of protective clothing	Not recommended for older adults
Sailing	Mainly for recreation and relaxation	Equipment and expense	Should be good swimmer

SPORT/EXERCISE/ ACTIVITY!	FITNESS BENEFITS	PARTICIPATION DISADVANTAGES	PRECAUTIONS
Skating			
Ice			
Roller	Excellent fitness activity if activity remains continuous	Contact injuries/ankle injuries	Good for all ages
Skiing			
Alpine	Muscular leg endurance	Cost/equipment	Need instruction
Nordic	One of the best all fitness activities	Equipment	Good for all ages
Water	Muscular strength/endurance	Boat/equipment	Need training
Slimnastics	Mainly flexibility, some muscle endurance		
Soccer	One of better all around fitness activities, except for goalie	Need team players	
Softball	Recreational/relaxation except for competitive leagues Low fitness developing sport	Need full team	Can pull muscles unless stretched through warm-up
Squash (handball)	Excellent fitness activity if competition is good and action is continuous	Facilities	Protect eyes
Surfing	Muscular fitness and coordination Low level aerobics	Safe ocean waters	Should be properly trained
Swimming	If follow training principles is one of best all around fitness activities, plus recreational and survival skills developed	Need safe swimming area	Learn to swim under a competent teacher
Scuba Diving	Depends upon activity level	Equipment/special training	Never dive alone
Springboard Diving	Muscle strength, coordination	Need proper board and training	Do not exceed present ability

SPORT/EXERCISE/ ACTIVITY	FITNESS BENEFITS	PARTICIPATION DISADVANTAGES	PRECAUTIONS
Tennis (singles, doubles, and table)	All can be fitness stimulating if training principles are followed, but usually is recreational and low aerobics	None: Good for all ages	
Track and Field Running (short) Running (long) Field events	Muscular fitness Aerobics fitness Muscular and skill fitness only		Training progressively Get in shape first
Volleyball	Muscular fitness, power, agility Minimal aerobics	Need court/team	Environment factors
Walking (backpacking)	Can be aerobic if duration is long, plus leg endurance	Need wooded trails	
Water Polo	Excellent all around fitness activity	Requires excellent water skills	Must be in superb condition
Weight Lifting Power lifting Body building	All can be effective in developing high level of muscular strength and muscular endurance	Need special equipment and facilities	Could be harmful to persons with special medical problems
Weight training	Circuit training can have aerobic effect if done properly		
Wrestling	Excellent all around fitness activity	Coaching required	Get in shape first
Yoga	Flexibility, relaxation, stress reduction and some muscle fitness	None: excellent for all ages	

Note: Individuals with special medical disorders or limitations should consult their physician prior to initiating serious participation in a sports or exercise program.

INDEX

ABOUT THE AUTHORS

Heinz W. Lenz is an Associate Professor in Physical Eduction in Annapolis, Maryland at the United States Naval Academy. He joined the faculty in 1957. He was born in Germany, lived in Italy and attended Ohio State and Columbia University, where he received the M.A. Degree. As chairperson of Personal Conditioning at the Naval Academy, he is primarily responsible for the physical fitness programs for the Brigade of Midshipmen. His experience includes coaching soccer and track at the Naval Academy. In addition to other responsibilities Professor Lenz conducts a physical fitness program for officers, faculty and staff at the United States Naval Academy.

Dr. John L. Murray is currently a Professor of Health and Physical Education at Catonsville Community College, Maryland. Formerly at that institution, he has held positions as Assistant to the President and Chairperson of the Health, Physical Education, Recreation and Athletic Division. As an administrator, he was largely responsible for implementing the highly successful Life Fitness Program and the well-known cardiac rehabilitation program PACE. His educational background includes degrees from West Chester State University (B.S.), Penn State University (M.S.) and the University of Maryland (PhD), with special emphasis in exercise physiology. In 1980 Dr. Murray authored a book titled, INFAQUATICS: TEACHING KIDS TO SWIM, a comprehensive and innovative guide to help parents teach their children to swim. Professor Murray is a former Marine, having served as a member of the U.S. Marine Corps drill team and guard unit during the Eisenhower presidency. He is not only a professional advocate of health, he actively participates in a variety of sport and fitness activities on a regular basis.